ALEXANDER CRUZ

Chromosomes and Genes

The Biological Basis of Heredity

NORTON LIBRARY
CONTEMPORARY SCIENCE PAPERBACKS

Reproduction and Man by Richard J. Harrison   N581
Reproduction and Environment by R. L. Holmes   N588
Chromosomes and Genes: The Biological Basis of Heredity
by Peo C. Koller   N587
Life: Its Nature, Origins, and Distribution
by Josephine Marquand   N589

P. C. KOLLER B.SC., PH.D., D.SC.
Professor of Cytogenetics, Chester Beatty Research Institute, London

Chromosomes and Genes

The Biological Basis of Heredity

The Norton Library

W · W · NORTON & COMPANY · INC ·
NEW YORK

Books That Live
The Norton imprint on a book means that in the publisher's
estimation it is a book not for a single season but for the years.
W. W. Norton & Company, Inc.

PRINTED IN THE UNITED STATES OF AMERICA

2 3 4 5 6 7 8 9 0

Dedicated to

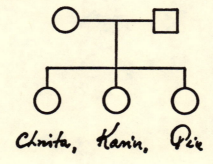

Chrita, Kanin, Pie

A new individual begins with the fusion of two microscopically tiny pieces of matter, the male and female sex cells. Together, these two cells contain all of the genes or instructions needed to control the correct development of a complete adult, whether plant or animal. That this can be so is one of the continuing wonders of life on earth, an event of staggering, near-miraculous complexity which is nevertheless enacted all around us every day.

N. SULLIVAN, 1967

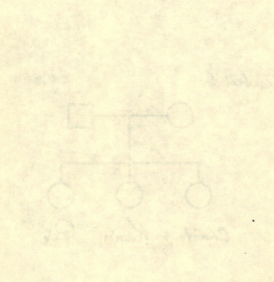

Preface

The fact that every human being is different poses a funda-
mental problem which concerns the transmission mechanism
of heredity between parents and offspring and the origin of
differences between them. During the past 50 years geneticists
answered many questions, and our progress towards a better
understanding of the mechanism of heredity became very
rapid indeed. There are today few scientific problems which
could be more exciting or which could attract more widespread
interest than those in the field of genetics.

The great advance has given us a new dimension; nowadays
we can not only discern genetic diversity of individuals, but
we are deciphering the genetic code and are exploring the
operation of the hereditary message on a molecular basis.
We are witnessing the emergence of 'molecular genetics'.
The new knowledge is increasing daily and has encouraged some geneticists and biochemists to believe that it
may become possible in the not too distant future for the
genetic heritage of individuals to be tailor-made by inducing change in the chemical structure of the basic units, the
genes.

The genes, which are located in the chromosomes of the cell,
existed in our ancestors before us and will persist in our
children's children after we have gone. They are responsible
for what we are. The physical sciences converged on the
chromosome, giving us new insights into its structure and
function; the mechanism of replication; the linear sequence of
its repeating units which form the genetic code, and the process by which the code is transcribed into specific protein
structure. The chromosomes and their genes occupy a central
position in the science of genetics and are acknowledged to be

the biological basis of human variation in health and disease. They are the subjects of our book.

The first part of the book aims to acquaint the reader with the basic principles of 'classical genetics', particularly with the experimental methods used to obtain the information which the formulation of these principles made possible. Without them, our generation might have been deprived of the exciting new discoveries which are amongst the greatest achievements of Man.

P. C. KOLLER

Contents

Preface **v**

1. The Control Centre of Cells 1
2. The Chromosome Basis of Heredity 36
3. Genes in Action 56
4. Cytogenetics: The Study of Chromosome Behaviour 97
5. The Genetic Load and Future of Man 127
   Appendix to the 1971 Edition 137
   Appendices 140
   Bibliography 142
   Acknowledgements 143
   Index 144

1. The Control Centre of Cells

The bodies of higher plants and animals including man are
made up of cells, all descended from the fertilised egg. Each
cell is a microcosm within which takes place many complex
chemical reactions fulfilling specific functions. We now know
that these activities are associated with definite sub-cellular
structures (organelles) within the cell and that their function is
under a centralised control. Our aim is to locate the site of
the control in the cell and to disclose the ways by which control
is exercised. The first task is to look at the structural anatomy
of the cell.

THE PHYSICAL ORGANISATION OF CELLS

The cell was discovered in 1665 by Robert Hooke; under his
home-made microscope he looked at a thin slice of cork and
saw a lattice-work structure made up of a multitude of small
compartments, like a honeycomb. Hooke called these little
compartments 'cells'. To him they appeared as empty boxes; in
reality, they were only the boundaries of dead cells. Over the
course of the following 300 years the complexity of the internal
organisation of cells gradually came to light, particularly after
the development of the electron microscope, which magnifies
many thousandfold.

The cell is capable of independent existence: it can grow,
move and multiply. Having these properties, the cell can be
considered to be the physical unit of life. Some of the lower
plants and animals remain as one cell throughout life; these
are called unicellular organisms to distinguish them from the
majority of plants and animals which are multicellular, being
made up of many cells. This fact was recognised as early as
1839, when Schwann referred to animals and plants as

1

'aggregates of cells which are arranged according to definite laws'. At the same time the two main components of the cell, *cytoplasm* and *nucleus*, had already been identified and described, but the classification of their chemical nature and function has only been accomplished in recent years.

The cytoplasm is composed of water (85–90%), proteins and lipids (8–12%), and a small amount of carbohydrates and inorganic substances, e.g. sodium, potassium. The most important of the cytoplasmic components are the proteins, the complex molecules made up of the nitrogen-containing amino acids. The character of the protein is determined by the number and sequence of the various amino acids in the molecule. The proteins are important cell components, they provide the basis for the structural organisation and functional role of cells. The lipids are fluid or semi-fluid substances, and include the fats and oils of plant or animal origin. They are essential constituents of various cell structures, e.g. cell membrane.

The cytoplasm also contains solid inclusions, or particles, called the 'organelles', some of which are no bigger than 1/100 000 of an inch and can be seen only through the electron microscope. The most important organelles are the mitochondria, endoplasmic reticulum (ergastoplasm), ribosomes (Plate I *above*), centrosomes including the centriole, microsomes, Golgi body, chloroplast and lysosomes. Some of these structures are shown diagrammatically in Fig. 1.

Mitochondria are rod-shaped or spherical structures and are present in practically every type of cell. They are composed of two membranes; the inner membrane is folded, providing a greater interior surface area. The number of mitochondria varies from cell to cell: some cell types have few, whilst others have many; the liver of the rat may have from 600–1000 which aggregate and form clusters.

Chloroplasts, which are only present in plant cells, are composed of parallel lamellae, or partitions, and surrounded by an outer membrane. This organelle contains the light-sensitive pigment, known as chlorophyll, which is responsible for the green colour of plants.

Endoplasmic reticulum (ER) is a three-dimensional network

of membranes forming a fine mesh of hollow sheets extending from the nucleus to the outer membrane of the cell. Being a labile system, its appearance changes rapidly.

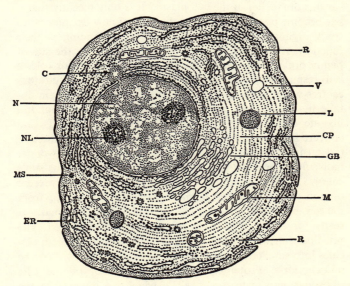

Fig. 1. *Diagram of a typical cell, based on what is seen in electron micrographs.* C = *centrosome (centriole);* N = *nucleus;* NL = *nucleolus;* MS = *microsome;* ER = *endoplasmic reticulum;* R = *ribosome;* V = *vacuole;* L = *lysosome;* CP = *cytoplasm;* GB = *Golgi body;* M = *mitochondria.*

Ribosomes are small, spherical-shaped 'granules' covering the outer surfaces of the ER.

Centriole is a small cylinder composed of parallel rods lying in a zone of clear cytoplasm (centrosome).

Microsomes are believed to be fragments of the ER containing the small granules (ribosomes).

Golgi body, first described by Camillo Golgi in 1898, is found in cells of tissues which secrete specific substances, e.g. pancreas, liver. It consists of four or five hollow, flat discs piled above each other, and the inner membranes are smooth.

Lysosomes are tiny sacs containing the digestive juices surrounded by a strong membrane.

A question that naturally arises is: what is the role of the
various organelles in the cytoplasm? It is only recently that it
has become possible, by the application of new techniques, to
study organelles and to get a better understanding of their
function. It is now known that mitochondria are the site of
highly organised enzyme systems which play a major role in
cell respiration; they can be considered as the respiratory
centres which account for the greatest portion of oxygen up-
take by the cell. By utilising the oxygen, the mitochondria
liberate energy from the broken-down raw materials and
convert it into chemical energy which is locked up in ATP
(adenosine triphosphate), often referred to as the 'wonder
molecule'. The ATP makes the cell independent of the sun's
energy. Another energy converter is the chloroplast, present
only in plants. Its green pigment traps the light-energy from
the sun, packages this energy into chemical form and makes it
ready for transportation to sites where it is required. The
principal function of the lysosomes is to destroy large molecules into smaller constituents which can then be used by the
mitochondria. Protein-synthesis is catered for by the ER,
ribosomes and microsomes, all of which are involved in the
process. The ER provides the surfaces for the chemical reactions as well as the pathways for transporting the synthesised
products, whilst the role of the Golgi body is believed to be
storage. The centrioles are the organising centres of the spindle
which is formed during cell division.

This brief summary of recent findings shows that the cytoplasmic organelles all play a part in the complex process of
cell metabolism and that their functions are interdependent.
Some are constructed to break down the raw materials which
enter the cell, others to extract and convert energy required to
build up substances essential for the life of the cell. These
functions are not carried out haphazardly; on the contrary,
they are well regulated.

The cell is surrounded by a membrane which permits
growth and movement; it has a peculiar double structure,

partly permeable to water. In the plant cells there is a more rigid 'wall' made of cellulose. Though cells have a definite boundary, neither the plasma membrane of animal cells nor the cellulose wall of plant cells should be looked upon as an envelope which isolates cells from each other. The electron microscope has revealed cytoplasmic connections between adjacent cells, thus binding them together into a community. It has been observed that at the region of cell contact substances diffuse freely from the interior of one cell to that of the next. Quite large molecules can cross the junctional surface membranes and can act as a signal for 'contact inhibition', when the cells which come into contact with each other stop moving and dividing. The exchange of information between cells is a major factor in the control of cell differentiation. The phenomenon of intercommunication between cells has been recently demonstrated by an electrical test: current of ions from a generator was passed through a microelectrode into the cell and the resulting voltage across the membrane of the 'injected' and adjacent cell was measured. It was found that a considerable fraction of the current introduced into liver cells of the rat passes to adjacent cells. It was also found that the ion flow was vastly greater between normal cells than between cancer cells. It is suggested that the electrical test for demonstrating intercommunication between cells may be used as a diagnostic test for cancer.

The complex chemical reactions which proceed and interact with each other in a continuous flux, all take place within the boundary of the cell. The size of cells shows tremendous variation; at one end of the scale there are the eggs of birds, the size of which is measured in centimetres; at the other end of the scale are the bacteria and viruses, whose size can be expressed in fractions of microns (see Appendix I).

When tissue cells are killed by chemical agents (e.g. alcohol or formalin) and then stained with special dyes, they show very great variation in shape; cells can be round, oblong, oval, needle- or spindle-shaped, etc. The shape of unicellular organisms, e.g. Amoeba, changes continuously.

The shape of cells is often dictated by pressure exerted from outside. It may, however, be the result of adaptation for a specific function. The cells of the skin are like paving stones pressed together to afford protection. The nerve cells are branched; they are part of the system which accepts and transmits messages through the cytoplasmic branches from cells to other cells many inches away. The blood cells and sperms being mobile, their shape is adapted to the function they have to serve. The red blood cells transport oxygen to other cells, whilst the white blood cells move through the body as scavengers.

THE CELL NUCLEUS

The nucleus, first seen in 1839 by the Englishman Brown, is a universal and essential part of cells. It is present in single-cell organisms, like the Amoeba, as well as in the cells of various tissues of higher animals and plants.

The best evidence that the nucleus is an essential cell component is provided by the unicellular Amoeba. When the nucleus is removed from the cytoplasm, the 'enucleated' portion of the Amoeba lives for a few days after the operation but its movement becomes slower and slower, it stops taking in food and eventually dies. So far no substitute has been discovered that can restore life to the 'enucleated' Amoeba, only when a nucleus from another Amoeba is transplanted into the enucleated portion will it be restored to full life. In another experiment the nucleus of the Amoeba was almost completely stripped of the surrounding cytoplasm and the drastically truncated Amoeba slowly grew back to its original size and became fully operative.

Amoebae can be killed by exposure to X-rays, which is the same method clinicians use to destroy cancer cells in the human body. When an Amoeba is exposed to a high dose of radiation, it stops moving, its cytoplasm undergoes rapid changes, and the animal dies. If, however, the nucleus of the irradiated Amoeba is replaced by a nucleus from a non-irradiated Amoeba, it soon recovers and carries on normal activity. When frog's eggs are enucleated their fate is the same as that of the enucleated Amoeba. If, however, such an egg cell is fertilised, the nucleus of the sperm enables the enucleated egg to multiply. Many experiments like those described above have been carried out using different cells, but the findings were always the same; removal of, or injury to, the nucleus impaired the life of the cell. It became obvious to the biologists that a healthy nucleus in the cell is essential for life.

The nucleus has another function in addition to that of maintaining life. The nature of this additional function becomes clear from the following experiment in which the green alga Acetabularia was used. It is a unicellular plant composed of three distinct parts, the base, stalk and cap, and the nucleus usually lies at the base of the stalk. This small plant has a great capacity for regeneration. When the cap of Acetabularia is cut away, a new one, like the one which was removed, will grow out at the end of the truncated stalk provided the base containing the nucleus was left intact. There are various kinds of green algae, such as *Acetabularia mediterranea* and *A. crenulata*, which are distinguishable by the different shape of their caps. It is possible to graft a piece of stalk from one alga on to the stalk of another from which the cap has been removed previously. The outcome of such grafting experiments is illustrated in Fig. 2.

When a stalk segment of *A. mediterranea* is grafted on to the nucleus-containing base of *A. crenulata*, it produces a cap which is characteristic of the species contributing the nucleus. Reversal of the grafting gives the same result. These experiments indicate that the shape of the cap is dictated by the portion of the cell which contains the nucleus. The obvious conclusion is that the nucleus, besides being necessary for the maintenance of life, has the capacity to imprint upon the cell a particular pattern of morphology and behaviour.

The grafting experiments with Acetabularia were carried out only a few years ago by Hämmerling, but experiments of a different kind which, nevertheless, led to a similar conclusion had already been made 60 years before by T. Boveri. He used two species of sea-urchins whose larvae differ in shape and size. The egg of the sea-urchin can be broken into several pieces when shaken strongly. Now, those portions which have no nucleus die. If, however, the enucleated egg-pieces are fertilised with sperms larvae develop, the shape and size of which is dictated by the sperm; it is always the same as that of

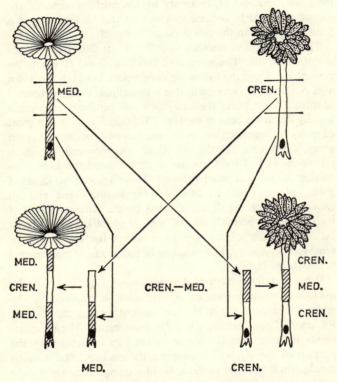

Fig. 2. *Hämmerling's grafting experiment between* Acetabularia mediterranea *and* crenulata.

the species which contributed the sperm. Boveri concluded that the nucleus of the sperm was responsible for determining the morphology of the sea-urchin larva.

These and several similar observations show that the nucleus, besides maintaining life, also controls the appearance and behaviour of the cell and the organism. The cap of

Acetabularia and the shape of the sea-urchin larva are two such examples of nuclear control.

The question naturally arises: what is it in the nucleus that governs the life and behaviour of cells? Under an ordinary microscope the appearance and structure of the nucleus is simple: it appears as a spherical-shaped vesicle surrounded by a porous semipermeable membrane, and contains smaller vesicles, the *nucleoli*. If the nucleus of a living cell is punctured with a fine needle, the contents diffuse into the cytoplasm of the cell without leaving a trace. Only when the cell is fixed and stained can we see some structures. These are fine filaments which form a network. This is referred to as the *chromatin* network, the Greek word indicating the ability of the filaments to absorb certain dyes. The network also contains several deeply stained bodies called the *chromocentres*. The contents of the nucleus have been analysed by the chemists, who found nucleic acids, proteins, lipids and traces of metals. The question was asked by many biologists: which of these constituents has the capacity to direct cell metabolism, to govern the interplay of chemical reactions and to control cell behaviour? We now know that it is the *nucleic acid* that has this power.

It was in 1868 that nucleic acid was first isolated by a young Swiss biochemist, Friedrich Miescher, from the nuclei of cells which appear in inflamed wounds, and from the sperms of salmon. The material thus obtained, however, was a mixture of nucleic acid and protein. Improvements in the method of extraction gradually resulted in obtaining nucleic acid in a purer state which could then be used by the chemists for more detailed study. It was shown to contain C, H, N, O and P. But it was only after 1930 that nucleic acid began really to interest biochemists and biologists. It soon became clear that there were two distinct varieties of this substance: one, found first only in plants, was shown to contain the sugar *ribose*, hence called 'ribose nucleic acid', or RNA for short; the other, first isolated from animal cells, was found to contain *deoxyribose* sugar and is called 'deoxyribose nucleic acid', or DNA.

During the last decade very intensive research has provided

further information about the distribution and behaviour of nucleic acid in various biological material. It has been established that this substance is present in every cell of higher organisms, as well as in the unicellular bacteria and viruses. The amount of nucleic acid present in the cells of different tissues of the same animal is fixed: e.g. in man, the cells of the liver, kidney, spleen and skin contain the same amount of nucleic acid. On the other hand, the quantity of nucleic acid in cells of different species is different: e.g. the amount of this substance in the cells of the mouse and in the cells of man differs. The basis of the specific stability of nucleic acid content in the different organisms will be discussed later. Since nucleic acid is present in every living organism, it can be postulated *a priori* that it must have a very important and specific role in the cell which no other cell structure could fulfil. The following experiments show that the ubiquitous nucleic acid is the substance which determines what cells should do.

The first example is provided by Pneumococcus, the unicellular bacterium which causes pneumonia. This bacterium exists in two forms: one is the virulent type causing the disease, the other is the harmless, or avirulent, type. The former can be killed by heating, and when mice are injected with the heat-killed bacteria they do not get ill but remain free of the disease as do mice which are injected with the harmless bacteria. Griffith in 1928 made a very important observation concerning the Pneumococcus. He injected a mixture of the heat-killed virulent and the living non-virulent bacteria into mice and found that some of the mice died of septicaemia. From these mice Griffith recovered the virulent-type bacteria, and concluded that the non-virulent bacteria were 'transformed' by the material which was present in the heat-killed virulent bacteria. Griffith died in 1941 during an air-raid in London, and did not know the elegant experiments reported in 1944 by a group of scientists in the United States. They extracted the nucleic acid from the virulent Pneumococcus bacteria, poured the substance into a test-tube which contained living non-virulent bacteria, and observed the 'transformation' of the harmless, avirulent bacteria into harmful virulent type *in vitro*. The transformation was revealed by injecting the bacteria which were in contact with the nucleic acid extract into mice, all of which developed pneumonia and died. The experiment verified Griffith's original interpretation that the 'transformation' was due to the material obtained from the dead virulent bacteria as well as identifying the 'transformation' substance. The problem of how and at which site the foreign nucleic acid becomes incorporated into the recipient bacteria will be discussed later.

In the second experiment, a virus was used which infects and kills bacteria; this particular bacterial virus is called *phage*. The most extensively studied phage is the one which infects the colon bacteria (*Escherichia coli*) of higher animals. The bacteriophage is like a tadpole in appearance having a head and tail (Fig. 3 and Plate I *below*). It is mostly composed of

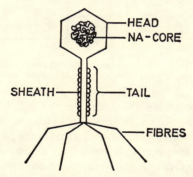

Fig. 3. *Diagram showing the structure of the bacteriophage.*

protein and the nucleic acid which forms the core in the head. The phages reproduce only within the bacterial cells they infect; when infection occurs, the phages anchor themselves by their tails to a suitable host bacterium. After that, the nucleic acid core is injected through the tail by an ingenious device into the cytoplasm of the bacterial cell where it multiplies and reconstitutes a new and complete phage which destroys the host bacterium. The coat of the virus remains outside as a ghost.

The process is illustrated in Fig. 4. By labelling the protein coat with radioactive atoms of sulphur, and the nucleic acid with radioactive tritium, it can be demonstrated that only the nucleic acid of the phage enters the bacterium.

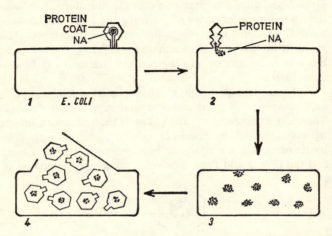

Fig. 4. *The infection of the colon bacterium* (E. coli) *with phage. (After Thompson & Thompson, 1966.)*

These experiments show that in the coli bacterium the nucleic acid carries the information which can be transferred from one bacterium to another and that in the phage it has the capacity to multiply and to reconstruct a new bacteriophage.

Exactly the same properties are expressed by the nucleus of cells in higher organisms. We know that a new individual arises from the fertilised egg, or ovum. The information by which development and differentiation proceeds from cell to cell, from tissue to tissue, from individual to individual, is packed into the nucleic acid of the fertilised egg. It seems obvious that this unique property must be embodied in some mysterious manner in the structural organisation of the nucleic acid. The question is: what kind of a chemical structure would be required which could store information and translate it into action without impairment of its stability?

THE SUBSTANCE OF HEREDITY

Research during the last two decades has lifted the veil which covered the mysteries of nucleic acid. First of all, it became clear that there is no specific plant or animal nucleic acid, the same substance being present in both. It was then discovered that DNA, the deoxyribose type of nucleic acid, is the substance which can be isolated from the cell nuclei, while RNA, the ribose nucleic acid, is regularly found in the cytoplasm of cells in large quantities. The former is endowed with the unique properties discussed previously, while the latter plays an intermediary role in protein synthesis. Recently, it was also discovered that in some viruses like tobacco mosaic virus and a few of the cancer-producing viruses, the RNA took over the role of DNA; in these organisms it became the substance of heredity which normally is the privilege of DNA.

The chemists found that nucleic acids (DNA as well as RNA) are very large molecules; they form long chains in which sub-units are repeated. These units are the 'nucleotides' which are composed of three parts: (i) base, (ii) sugar and (iii) phosphoric acid.

The bases are of two main types, purines and pyrimidines, composed of carbon and nitrogen atoms in varying numbers. The pyrimidine bases have a single five-membered ring structure, to which are attached other atoms forming three varieties of pyrimidines: cytosine (C) and thymine (T) in the DNA; cytosine (C) and uracil (U) in the RNA molecule. The purines have a double ring structure, because another five-membered ring is added to the pyrimidine ring thus increasing the number of carbon and nitrogen atoms. There are two main purine bases, adenine (A) and guanine (G), which are present in both DNA and RNA. The chemical analysis has shown that RNA differs from DNA in its sugar and base composition; in RNA the pyrimidine base thymine (T) is replaced with uracil (U). In the uracil molecule the methyl group (CH_3) of the thymine is absent.

The chemical structures of the four bases and the two types of sugar are shown in Fig. 5. The combination of one base,

THE BASES

THE PURINES

GUANINE

ADENINE

THE PYRIMIDINES

NH₂

THYMINE

CYTOSINE

THE SUGARS

CH₂OH   OH

OH

DEOXYRIBOSE

CH₂OH   OH

RIBOSE

A. NUCLEOTIDE

PHOSPHATE

$O = P - O - CH_2$

ADENINE

DEOXYRIBOSE

OH

Fig. 5. *Chemical structure of the various bases, sugars and nucleotides.*

one sugar and one phosphate molecule forms one nucleotide unit. In the long chain of DNA or RNA, many thousands or millions of such nucleotides are joined together by sugar–phosphate linkages and form the polynucleotide chain:

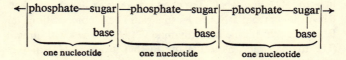

The application of new and refined techniques enabled the chemists to measure the amount of DNA in tissues and cells and the relative proportion of the bases present in their DNA samples. The findings were extremely interesting and can be summarised as follows:

(i) the amount of DNA extracted from different tissues of the same animal is the same;

(ii) the base composition in a particular DNA molecule is constant; the amount of adenine equals the amount of thymine (A = T), and similarly the amount of guanine equals the amount of cytosine (G = C);

(iii) the base ratio (A + T) : (G + C) in the DNA taken from different tissues or cells of the same animals is fixed, i.e. it is always the same;

(iv) the base ratio in the DNA of animals of different species, differs. Some of these findings are well illustrated in Table 1.

Table 1. *Base composition in the DNA.*

Source of DNA	Purine Bases		Pyrimidine Bases		Base Ratio $\dfrac{A + T}{G + C}$
	Adenine	*Thymine*	*Guanine*	*Cytosine*	
BACTERIA					
Micrococcus	0·15	0·15	0·35	0·35	0·41
E. coli	0·25	0·25	0·25	0·25	1·00
MAMMALIAN TISSUE					
Calf thymus	0·29	0·28	0·21	0·22	1·32

These observations were important. They indicated that the structure and organisation of DNA molecules must be arranged according to a common pattern. Although we had much information concerning the chemical composition and base ratios in DNA, it could not tell us how the component units are arranged in the giant polynucleotide chains so that DNA could satisfy the requirements of heredity. What was needed was a three-dimensional model of the DNA.

Progress towards this aim was made by applying X-ray diffraction analysis. This method is used very successfully to disclose the arrangement of molecules in crystals. When X-rays are passed through molecules, the atoms in the molecules deflect the X-ray particles, which produce a 'diff-raction pattern' on the photographic plate. The pattern of spots is used by experts to produce a three-dimensional arrangement of the atoms within the molecule. By applying this method, the complex structure of proteins such as myo-globin in muscle and haemoglobin in red blood cells has been disclosed. This was the technique which M. H. F. Wilkins and his colleagues in King's College applied to DNA. They looked at DNA collected from various sources, and found that in spite of the different base ratios the diffraction patterns were identical and the nucleotide bases were arranged perpendic-ularly to the backbone of the polynucleotide chains.

The problem was how to fit the bases to the sugar–phosphate backbone in view of the fact that the purine bases are larger than the pyrimidine bases and that the distance between adjacent nucleotides is the same. The solution of the problem is due to J. D. Watson and F. H. C. Crick, who in 1953 produced a molecular model of DNA in which the biochemical and physical properties of this substance could be reconciled. They assumed that the DNA molecule is composed of two chains of polynucleotide in which the bases are linked together by hydrogen bonds (Fig. 6). The different shape of the bases and the angle at which these are joined to each other and linked to the sugar molecule led Watson and Crick to suggest that the two polynucleotide chains are twisted around each other, forming a double helix like a spiral staircase in which the base to base attachments represent the series of steps. According to this model the adenine is specifically paired with thymine, and guanine with cytosine. The Watson-Crick model of DNA is illustrated in Fig. 7, in which the specific pairing of bases A—T and G—C is indicated.

Can the model cater for the great diversity and variability of living things? How can it store the enormous quantity of information required for development and differentiation of an organism? The structural composition of DNA satisfies these requirements, because the number of possible variations in the sequence of the bases is *limitless*. In the human cell the amount of DNA, if arranged into one continuous thread,

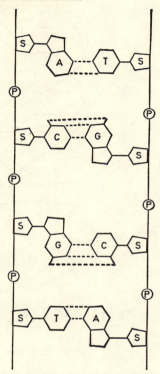

Fig. 6. *The molecular structure of the two polynucleotide strands in which the bases are linked together.*

would be only three feet long, yet it contains all the information which dictates our similarities and differences!

THE VEHICLE OF DNA IN THE CELL

It has already been stated that DNA is present in the nucleus of all cells of an organism in the same amount, while RNA, the other moiety of nucleic acid, is found in the cytoplasm and varies greatly in amount from cell to cell. This finding is the most powerful argument that DNA is the substance of heredity. The question is: what is the basis of the constancy of

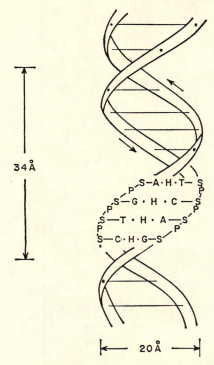

Fig. 7. *The Watson-Crick model of DNA molecule; the two sugar–phosphate chains (S—P—S) are held together by H bonds between the bases of the two chains and form a double helix.* A = *adenine;* T = *thymine;* G = *guanine;* C = *cytosine;* S = *sugar;* P = *phosphate group. (After Watson & Crick, 1953.)*

DNA in the cells as well as in the species and how is this constancy maintained?

The overwhelming evidence indicates that the nuclear structures responsible for the stability and constancy of the DNA are the *chromosomes*. In most cells, they are hidden in the chromatin network of the nucleus but become visible during the division of cells. This process, called *mitosis*, was observed in 1848 by Hofmeister. He watched a living plant cell under the microscope and made drawings of what he saw. Hofmeister noted the appearance of small rod-like bodies moving about the cytoplasm, crowding in the centre of the cell and then moving apart to form two groups each of which became a separate nucleus. Hofmeister's report was the first description of cell division, the true significance of which, however, was only recognised 30 years later when it became possible to study mitosis in fixed and suitably stained cells. The rod-like bodies of Hofmeister were given the name 'chromosomes', the Greek word indicating their affinity to certain dyes when the cell is fixed.

Mitosis is the process by which cells multiply and the body of higher organisms is built up. It is also the precise apparatus

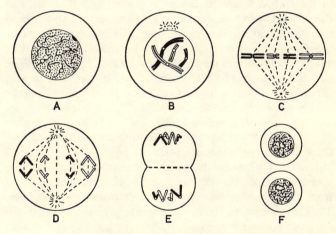

Fig. 8. *Diagram showing the various stages of mitosis: A = interphase; B = prophase; C = metaphase; D = anaphase; E = telophase. Two chromosome pairs shown. (After Thompson & Thompson, 1966.)*

which ensures that the cells derived by this process receive the same amount of DNA as the parental cell had. The various stages of mitosis are illustrated in Fig. 8.

The first sign of cell division is indicated by the condensation of the nuclear network which resolves into the chromosomes appearing as distinct strands, some showing a double structure. This stage is called *prophase*. During this stage the 'strands' become thicker, and after the dissolution of the nuclear envelope, spread out in the cytoplasm revealing that they are composed of two strands lying closely parallel or twisting around each other (Plate II *above*). The sister strands are the *chromatids*, which are held firmly together at one spot, the *centromere*. While the chromosomes are organised into definite structures, the two small bodies of *centrioles*, lying outside the nucleus, separate from each other and migrate towards opposite poles in the cell where they begin to form the spindle, composed of contractile protein fibres. By using the technique of microsurgery G. C. Hoskins of Texas University in the United States succeeded in pulling spindle fibres and their associated chromosomes out of the nucleus and studied the effect of various enzymes on them. His finding suggests that the fibres consist of strands of DNA and of protein, their strength being due to the DNA, their elasticity to protein. The mitotic spindle can be demonstrated only by special treatment (Plate II *right*); in most cells fixed and stained for studying the chromosomes the spindle is invisible. The contracted chromosomes orientate themselves on the equatorial plate in the centre of the cell and link up at their centromere with the spindle fibres. This stage is the *metaphase*.

The separation of the sister chromatids takes place in *anaphase*. The chromatids become free at the centromere, and from this time on they are called daughter chromosomes. They move towards the opposite poles, where they form the daughter nucleus losing their visible identity. The aggregation of chromosomes into the two nuclei is followed by the division of the cytoplasm of the cell into two daughter cells. This stage is called *telophase*, the end of which is marked by the loosening up of the condensed chromosomes into a fine chromatin network in the nucleus. Another division may follow. The length of 'interphase' (formerly called 'resting stage') between successive divisions varies: it can last a few hours, several months, or even years. Some cells never divide again, e.g. the nerve cells.

One might wonder if the stages of mitosis observed in cells killed by fixative agents and stained by dyes do represent the sequence of events actually occurring in dividing cells. The introduction of phase contrast microscopy into cytology has made it possible to study living cells. In suitable cells, the mitotic process has been filmed by this technique and the observations verified the findings made on cells which were killed at various stages of division.

The mitotic chromosomes, as we see them on the equatorial plate, are solid structures in which the double helix of the DNA molecule forms only the core, or backbone. It is known that the chromosome contains a large amount of basic protein, which is mostly histone. The presence of DNA in the chromosome is disclosed by the Feulgen reaction. This consists of two steps. First, the purines of DNA are removed by hydrolysis, which opens up the deoxyribose ring; secondly, the aldehyde group which has been formed reacts with the Schiff's reagent and gives a coloured complex. When the DNA content of the chromosome is removed, the reaction cannot take place, and the chromosome is left colourless. This test can be performed by applying an enzyme which is very specific in its action, disrupting only the structural organisation of the DNA, and which for this reason it is called the DNA-ase. When this enzyme was applied to the substance extracted from the virulent Pneumococcus, it lost its transforming property, indicating that the genetic instruction was in the DNA.

The chromosomes exhibit great differences in length, shape and number (see Plates III, IV, V, VI, VII, & XII *above*). The 'giant' chromosomes in the salivary gland of the fruit fly Drosophila (Plate XI *above*) are a few millimetres long, while some chromosomes of birds are not more than 0·5 microns. The most common size range, however, lies between 1 and 15 microns. It seems that the length of the chromosomes is adapted to the space available for their movement within the cell; a very long chromosome in a small cell would find great difficulty in moving to the pole and in being incorporated into the daughter nucleus.

The shape depends on the location of the centromere in the

chromosome, which is usually indicated by a constriction. Accordingly, the chromosome can be telocentric (or acrocentric), subtelocentric, submetacentric or metacentric, as shown in Fig. 9. A metacentric chromosome has two arms of

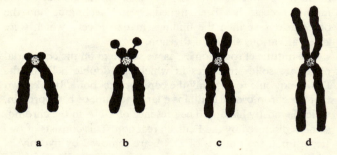

a   b   c   d

Fig. 9. *Various chromosome shapes:* a = *telocentric;* b = *subtelocentric with satellites;* c = *submetacentric;* d = *metacentric.*

equal length. Submetacentric and subtelocentric chromosomes have arms of different lengths; the short arm can be divided into two segments, the distal one being attached with a long constriction to the other region adjacent to the centromere. The short chromosome segment is referred to as the satellite. The telocentric chromosome has only one arm, and the centromere is positioned at the end or very near the end of such a chromosome.

The shape is a very important feature by which individual chromosomes in a chromosome set or complement can be recognised. The centromere is also responsible to some extent for the movement of chromosomes in the mitotic spindle. If a chromosome segment is broken away from the centromere, its active mobility is lost.

The number of chromosomes varies between species, but it is the same in each individual belonging to the same species. Thus every normal human being has 46 chromosomes in the body cells, every mouse has 40 chromosomes. A selected list of chromosome numbers in different species is given in Table 2.

Table 2. *Chromosome number in various species of animals and plants.*

Species	Number	Species	Number
Copepode-crab	6	Mouse	40
Drosophila	8	Rat	42
Broad bean	12	Rabbit	44
Garden pea	14	Man	46
Onion	16	Deer mouse	48
Corn	20	Striped skunk	50
Opossum	22	Spectacled bear	52
Tomato	24	Cebus monkey	54
Mink	30	Donkey	62
Fox	34	Horse	64
Pig	38	Aulacantha (Protozoa)	1600

The chromosomes of a cell can be arranged in pairs according to length and shape. There is, however, an exception. Commonly in the male sex of the mammals, two chromosomes in the chromosome set do not match. In man, one of these chromosomes is short, and as it is present only in the male sex it is referred to as the male sex-chromosome and designated as the Y chromosome (Plates VII *above*, and XI *below*); the other is a medium-sized submetacentric chromosome which has a matching partner in the female sex. This chromosome is the female sex-chromosome and is called the X chromosome. The other 22 pairs of chromosomes are not concerned with sex, they are the *autosomes*. The chromosome constitution of the two sexes of man therefore can be expressed as 22 pairs of autosomes and XY sex chromosome in the male, and 22 pairs of autosomes and XX sex chromosome in the female, the total number in both complements thus being 46 chromosomes.

The chromosomes of man have been classified and divided into definite groups by cytologists according to length and shape seen in the metaphase stage. The chromosome pairs are numbered from 1 to 22 in decreasing order of size and divided into seven groups represented by the letters A to G. The X chromosome is included in group C with chromosomes 6–12, while the Y chromosome is included in group G with chromosomes 21 and 22. The classification of the 22 autosomal chromosomes and the X and Y sex chromosomes is illustrated in Fig. 10.

Every cell in the human body contains 46 chromosomes except the sex cells – sperm and egg, or ovum – called *gametes*. The sex cells contain only 23 chromosomes, i.e. half the number present in the body cells. In the latter, each chromosome type is represented *twice*, in the gametes each type is *single*. The 46 chromosome-containing cells are called *diploid* ($2n = 46$), to distinguish them from the gametes in which the chromosome number is *haploid* ($n = 23$). The constancy of chromosome constitution in the cells of the body corresponds with the stability of the DNA content in the nucleus of the body cells. In the gametes, the quantity of DNA present is half of that measured in body cells. These facts are further evidence that the bearers of the hereditary substance are the chromosomes.

In the past few years many studies of chromosomes, particularly those concerning mammalian chromosomes, including man, have been made. It is hoped that by such studies some insight might be gained into evolutionary processes. The close association of chromosomes with the genetic constitution which is represented by the DNA, make them valuable as markers of genetic characters. Though the same features of chromosomes in different species do not necessarily indicate that they carry the same genetic information, the strong similarities observed in *karyotypes*, i.e. in the arrangement of metaphase chromosomes in closely related species, are considered to be of special significance from the evolutionary aspect. Such comparative studies led to the conclusion that on the basis of chromosome morphology only, the northern chimpanzee is most closely related to man; the pigmy chimpanzee, gorilla and the Asiatic ape (orang-outang) would follow. All the great apes mentioned have 48 chromosomes, two more than man. The similarities and dissimilarities in the chromosome constitution are shown in Table 3. It can be seen that the northern chimpanzee has one pair of large acrocentric chromosomes more than man. The gorilla, believed by many people to be the nearest relative of man, has a

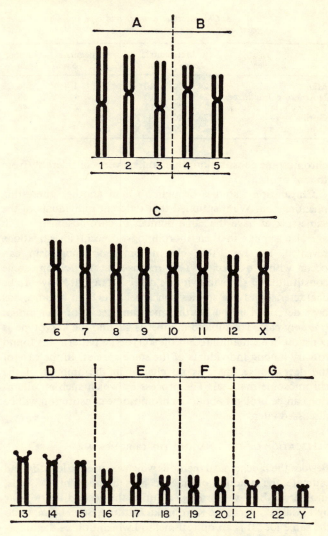

Fig. 10. *Schematic representation of the various chromosome types in the human karyotype.*

Table 3. *Chromosome number and type in man and in the great apes.*

| Species | Metacentric | | Acrocentric | | Number |
	Large	Small	Large	Small	2n
Man	24 + X	10	6	4 + Y	46
Northern chimpanzee	24 + X	10	8	4 + Y	48
Pigmy chimpanzee	24 + X	12	8	2 + Y	48
Gorilla	24 + X	6 + Y	12	4	48
Orang-outang	22 + X	6 + Y	16	2	48

chromosome constitution which differs very considerably from that of man.

Chromosome studies brought to light another interesting phenomenon. We mentioned that different individuals of the same species have the same number of chromosomes, which are also similar in their morphology. Recent investigations revealed, however, that chromosomal polymorphism can occur within a species. This means that the chromosome constitution of some individuals differs from that known to be characteristic of the species concerned. Such an instance has been described in the North American species of deer mouse (*Peromyscus*). The diploid number is 48, and the karyotype is constant in each animal, but the karyotype pattern was found to vary among individuals of the same species. In the case of the deer mouse, there is no change in the amount of the chromosome material. The process by which such an alteration can be brought about in chromosome constitution will be discussed later.

REPLICATION OF THE DNA AND THE CHROMOSOME

Besides the biochemical methods which are used to identify and estimate the amount of nucleic acid components of cells, another method was developed during the Second World War by T. Caspersson at the Karolinska Institute, Stockholm, to do the same job. It is an optical method which utilises the differential absorption of light at specific wavelengths by chemical substances. Instead of visible light ordinarily employed in conventional microscopy, Caspersson used ultraviolet as the source of light; the great advantage is that ultraviolet is strongly absorbed at a characteristic wavelength by nucleoproteins of the living cell. The 'ultraviolet microscope' is a useful and convenient tool to measure the amount and distribution of nucleic acid in the cell nucleus and chromosomes.

It was soon discovered, with the help of this instrument, that cells during interphase undergo cyclic changes in respect of their nucleic acid content. The ultraviolet microscope revealed that just before the onset of mitosis the amount of DNA is doubled. Furthermore, it was also found that the total amount of DNA in the prophase and metaphase chromosomes was twice as much as the amount characteristic of the species. These findings indicate that during interphase prior to mitosis not only do the chromosomes replicate, but their genetic material, the DNA, does the same. The question is how the complex DNA molecule replicates.

The structural organisation of DNA, as suggested by Watson and Crick, is well adapted to 'self-replication'. According to the model, the sequence of bases of one polypeptide DNA chain determines the position of the bases on the other chain; adenine (A) must pair with thymine (T), and guanine (G) with cytosine (C). The two DNA chains are complementary. Thus the sequence of bases

$$—A—T—G—A—C—$$

in one strand demands the sequence

$$—T—A—C—T—G—$$

in the other to form the double helix:

$$—A—T—G—A—C—$$
$$| \quad | \quad | \quad | \quad |$$
$$—T—A—C—T—G—$$

The first step in the process of replication is the unwinding of the double helix; this occurs by breaking the hydrogen bonds between the nucleotide bases. The single DNA strands with their nucleotides sticking out on the sugar–phosphate backbone serve as a mould or *template* on which a new complementary DNA strand is constructed, following the 'rule of base-pairing'. From the substances present in the cell free nucleotides composed of base sugar–phosphate molecules are built up in the cytoplasm, and are transported to the template DNA, where the base component of the free nucleotide joins by H-bond to the appropriate base of the template or 'parent' DNA. The sugar–phosphate groups of the adjacent nucleotides are connected and form the continuous backbone of the new, or 'daughter', DNA strand. The new DNA strand is identical to the strand which it replaces. The process of replication is shown diagrammatically in Fig. 11.

That the DNA molecule could make *new* DNA was beautifully demonstrated by A. Kornberg in the United States. He mixed together a large number of free nucleotides in a test-tube, these were the raw materials to which he added natural DNA extracted from the colon bacteria and a special enzyme required for other duties in the construction of the DNA. The natural DNA of the bacteria acted as the template on which the free nucleotides were moulded into the new DNA strands. Kornberg also demonstrated that the new DNA strands were capable of carrying on the synthesis of other strands in the same way as they do in the living cell. Kornberg received the Nobel Prize in 1959 for discovering DNA polymerase, which made possible the synthesis of new DNA in the test-tube. (Appendix II.) The proof, however, was lacking till recently that the new DNA was an accurate copy of the template DNA, since it was biologically inactive although it had the physical and chemical properties of natural DNA. A *biologically active* copy of DNA was recently produced by Kornberg and his associates, their achievement being greeted by the popular press as 'creation of life in a test-tube'. As the synthesis still required two substances, the catalysing enzyme DNA polymerase and the template DNA which are found only in living cells, it is not correct to refer to it as 'creation of life in a test-tube'. Kornberg's discovery is extremely important. It shows that the structural organisation of DNA, as it is

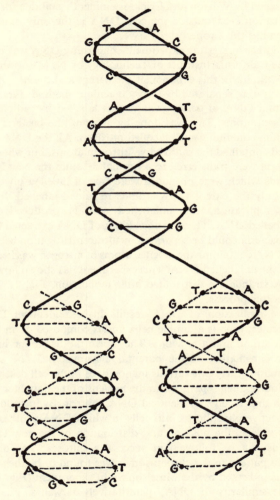

Fig. 11. *Diagram showing the replication of the DNA molecule.*

envisaged by Watson and Crick, is eminently suitable for self-replication even outside the cell. DNA is the only molecule which has this property!

Another interesting experiment concerning DNA was made at the California Institute of Technology by N. Meselson and F. W. Stahl. In this experiment the parent and the new DNA strands were separated by a very ingenious method. First, the parental DNA of colon bacteria was labelled by radioactive nitrogen atoms. This was done by growing the bacteria in a medium containing such labelled nitrogen. All the DNA produced contained the radioactive nitrogen atoms, but when the bacteria were transferred to a normal medium the new DNA strands which were produced were free of labelled nitrogen, and only the parent DNA strands remained labelled. In the next replication, the unlabelled strands produced only unlabelled DNA. These various kinds of DNA extracted from the bacteria could be separated by ultracentrifugation because the DNA containing the labelled atoms of nitrogen was heavier than the unlabelled DNA. This experiment has shown how the DNA strands are distributed after replication. Fig. 12 illustrates this process.

The replication of DNA results in two identical DNA molecules; each is a double helix and is composed of an 'old' DNA strand and a new one. They form the backbone in the sister chromatids of the parental chromosome. The sister chromatids carry out various manoeuvres in the cell described previously, then separate into the nucleus of the daughter cells which thus receive an identical DNA content. By introducing radioactive phosphorus into cells in which DNA synthesis is taking place, the position and distribution of the new DNA strands can be followed in successive mitoses. The distribution pattern in the chromosomes was found to be the same as was indicated by the Meselson-Stahl experiment (Fig. 12).

The similarity of DNA, quantitatively as well as qualitatively, suggests that the genetic information received by the daughter cells is also identical. Two observations may be mentioned to show that this is the case. When the daughter cells of a fertilised egg of the newt are separated from each other, they continue to divide and develop into two adult newts; both adults are always of the same sex, have similar colour patterns in their skin, and in other respects they behave

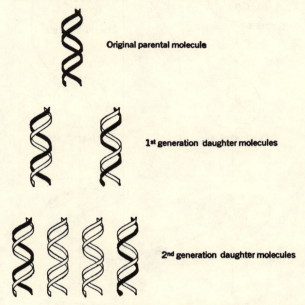

Original parental molecule

1st generation daughter molecules

2nd generation daughter molecules

Fig. 12. *The Meselson-Stahl experiment; by using radio-isotope labelling, the distribution of the old and newly synthesised DNA molecules is demonstrated. The parental polynucleotide chains are shown in black, the newly formed strands in white. (After Meselson & Stahl, 1958.)*

as identical twins. A similar experiment was performed by E. P. Volpe and R. G. McKinnel, who used cells from the developing embryo of the frog (Fig. 13). The nucleus from two cells lying in the outer layer of the blastula was isolated and transplanted into eggs from which the nucleus was previously removed. The artificially 'fertilised' eggs divided and produced two normal adults which were similar in appearance. These investigators exchanged pieces of skin between the animals and found that the skin pieces were accepted and became

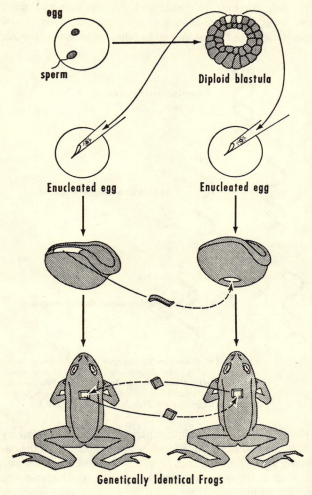

Fig. 13. *Transfer of nuclei from cells of the blastula into enucleated egg cells, followed by normal development; the acceptance of skin grafts shows that the frogs are genetically identical.*

incorporated into the skin of the recipient. The mutual acceptance of skin or other tissues between two animals is the best
evidence that they have the same genetic constitution. In the
experiment with the fertilised egg of the newt, the two identical
twin newts were derived from the two daughter cells of the
fertilised egg. In Volpe and McKinnel's experiment, the nuclei
of cells which were used were the result of several divisions
occurring after fertilisation, yet the frogs were identical. This
fact shows the process of mitosis to be a very precise mechanism which ensures the stability and constancy of the genetic
material from cell to cell.

THE LINK BETWEEN GENERATIONS

The cells of the body of higher organisms are descendants of
one cell: the fertilised egg. This ancestor of all cells has been
produced by the union of male and female gametes – sperm
and egg, or ovum. The union of these cells is called fertilisation and marks the beginning of a new organism.

In order that a species can remain in existence, its members
must reproduce themselves and bring forth a new generation
in an unending succession. The continuation of the species is
ensured by the ability of the adult individuals of the new
generation to produce gametes like their parents which will
unite at fertilisation and initiate another cycle of reproduction.
The gametes are the sole link between generations.

If the number of chromosomes in the gametes was the same
as in the other cells of the body, their union would produce a
new individual who would have *twice* as many chromosomes
as his or her parents had. In man, infants would be born with
92 chromosomes instead of 46; individuals of the next generation would have 184 chromosomes in their body cells, and by
the end of the tenth generation the number would be 23 332!
Such a happening is, however, prevented by a special division
which reduces the diploid number of chromosomes to half in
the gametes; in man it is reduced from 46 to 23. This occurs by
a process called *meiosis*; it consists of two nuclear divisions
during which the chromosomes divide only once. Meiosis is
often referred to as reduction division. Fig. 14 shows the chief

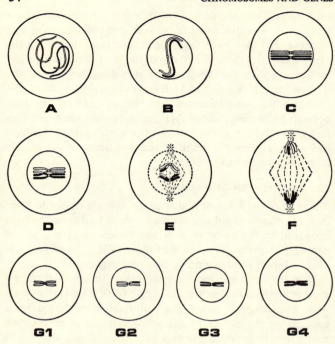

Fig. 14. *Diagram shows the various stages of the first meiotic, or reduction, division. The pairing of homologous chromosomes (B and C) is followed by chiasma formation (D) which results in an exchange of segments between chromatids (G2 and G3).*

features of meiosis; in the diagram we illustrate the behaviour of one pair of chromosomes only.

The most important event occurs during prophase, which is longer in duration than in mitosis and is grossly modified. The chromosomes are still single strands when they become visible, and they are still single when they associate and form a chromosome pair. The homologous chromosomes, i.e. those which are similar in length and shape, lie very close to each other, and only when the pairing is completed do they divide into two chromatids. At the same time, the chromatids of the homologous chromosomes exchange parts at one or at several points; the configuration produced by the exchange is the *chiasma*, named after the Greek letter chi = x. Following this event, the paired chromosomes become shorter in length, and when the nuclear membrane disappears the associated chromosomes move to the equatorial plate of the cell and attach themselves to the spindle. During anaphase the partners of the chromosome pairs separate and migrate to the opposite poles. With this event the reduction of chromosome number is completed; in our diagram each pole has one chromosome only instead of two.

The second meiotic division usually follows without an interphase; the chromosomes undergo normal mitosis. After the completion of the second meiotic division the cells stop dividing and mature into gametes: sperm or egg. While in the male all the four cells formed develop into sperms, in the female only one cell matures into an egg, the other three cells (polar bodies) die.

The presence of half the number of chromosomes in the gametes explains why the chemists could find only half the amount of DNA in these cells. The diploid chromosome number as well as the normal amount of DNA is restored in the fertilised egg by the mixing together of the chromosomes of the haploid sperm and egg. The chromosomes of the fertilised egg and its descendant cells can be sorted out into individual pairs, one member of which is of paternal, the other of maternal origin.

Meiosis is a very important event in sexually reproducing species, for two reasons: it maintains the chromosome constitution characteristic of the species through the generations by reducing the chromosome number in the gametes, and it brings about the final mixing of the parental hereditary material by the exchange of parts between homologous chromosomes.

2. The Chromosome Basis of Heredity

The observations we presented in the preceding chapter show very convincingly that the most important and essential part of the cell is the nucleus. We illustrated with examples that it maintains life and dictates the behaviour and morphology of the cell as well as the organism. In the DNA we identified the material basis of all these activities, described its molecular construction and the process by which its stability is maintained. It was shown that in this process the chromosomes are the vehicle of DNA and are responsible for its distribution from cell to cell and from individual to individual.

The next task is to demonstrate that the 'Laws of Heredity' rest on the chromosome mechanism and that all characteristics of the individual can be traced to the DNA as the ultimate source.

THE LAWS OF MENDEL

Differences amongst plants and animals were already noticed by man of prehistoric time. The writings of the Greek and Roman philosophers show that they were well aware of the differences and similarities between parents and their offspring and that they enquired into the cause. Their discourse on this subject, however, is only fanciful speculation. Even the theories of the great scientists of the last century, like Weismann and Darwin, could not account for the fact that not all features of the parents appear in their children.

The real understanding of heredity, the process by which the physical and mental characteristics of parents are transmitted to their offspring, is due to the Augustinian monk, Gregor Mendel. The experiments with the ordinary garden pea by which he established the principles of heredity took 13 years and were carried out in the small garden of the monastery. The two communications containing his work were read before the Natural Science Society of Brünn in 1865. Mendel's papers show him to be one of the great men of science. The description of the experiments is factual, concise and clear. The experiments themselves are flawless in design and perfect in execution, but, most of all, the interpretation of the experimental findings declares him to be a genius. Mendel supported his idea by evidence of a quantitative statistical kind which was also novel in its presentation. The theoretical model he produced predicted the properties and behaviour of the physical mechanism of heredity.

In order to realise the significance of the Mendelian principles, the experiments on which they were established will be described in detail.

The first law

In the monastery garden surrounded by the cloister, Mendel grew 22 varieties of peas, some tall, some dwarf; others had round seeds or wrinkled ones; the flowers of some were purple, others were white, etc. He crossed the different varieties by removing the stamens from the flower of one and fertilising the ovum of this plant with pollen (the male gamete) and covering each ·bloom so handled with a tiny linen bag to prevent fertilisation by other pollen. When the pods ripened, Mendel collected large numbers of seeds and planted them in the following spring. The results of such crossing, or 'hybridisation', may be best illustrated by using Mendel's own data which he obtained by crossing pea plants with tall stems with the dwarf variety. All the plants of the first generation (or F_1) from this crossing had tall stems. Mendel allowed these tall plants to self-pollinate by covering the blooms with linen bags. In the autumn he collected the seeds and sowed them in the next spring. From more than 1000 seeds sown, Mendel got 787 tall plants and 277 dwarf plants, the ratio being nearly 3:1.

Similar crossing experiments, in which other varieties were used, gave the same results; Mendel found that the ratio of the two varieties of the grandparents in the second generation was always 3:1. What could be the explanation for this regularity? The consistent results led Mendel to assume the presence of two 'factors' in each plant which influenced a character, e.g. the length of stem, the shape of seed, the colour of flower, etc. He postulated that the 'factor' of the character which appears in the first generation must be *dominant* over the 'factor' present in the other parent. The latter 'factor', and the character which is influenced by this 'factor', Mendel called *recessive*. Thus the 'factor' of tall stem is dominant, and the 'factor' responsible for the dwarf stem is recessive. The former is indicated by a capital letter T, the latter with a corresponding small letter t. By using these symbols, the experiment with the tall and dwarf peas can be written:

$$TT \times tt = \text{(Parent plants)}$$
$$|$$
$$Tt \quad = \text{(F}_1 \text{ hybrid)}$$

From the result of the self-pollination of Tt plants, Mendel deduced that the T and t factors must have been separated or segregated in the first generation plants, producing two kinds of gametes in equal number, one with the dominant T and the other with the recessive t factor. During self-pollination the union of gametes is governed by chance; consequently, the proportion of the various plant types due to recombination of the gametes with T or t factors could be *predicted*. Fig. 15 illustrates the segregation and recombination of T and t factors and shows the ratio of the two types in the second generation. The diagram also reveals that the tall plants are not uniform as regards the composition of their two factors: $\frac{1}{3}$ of them has two T factors, while the other $\frac{2}{3}$ has one T and one t. According to this scheme, it can be expected that the first kind of tall plants (TT) when self-pollinated would produce only tall plants; the second group of tall plants (Tt) when self-pollinated would yield both tall and dwarf peas in the ratio of 3:1. The dwarf plants having two t factors would produce only dwarfs. Planting the seeds of the second generation, Mendel obtained plants according to the expectation, and drew the conclusion that factors determining the different characters,

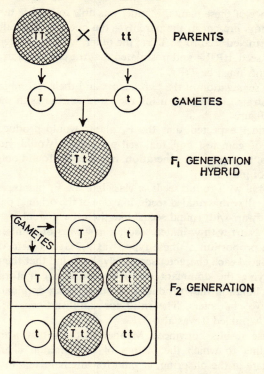

Fig. 15. *Mendel's first law, illustrated in the cross between tall (T) and dwarf (t) pea plants.*

e.g. length of stem, colour of flower, segregate from each other in the first generation offspring. This became known as the first law of Mendel.

The second law

Mendel made other crosses in which the parent plants differed in more than one character. In one such experiment he crossed a tall pea plant which produced wrinkled seeds with a dwarf variety which had round seeds, and obtained hybrids which were all tall and produced only round seeds. From the ap-

pearance of these plants, Mendel was able to deduce the kind
of factors present in the parents – the one with the tall stem
and wrinkled seed to be TTrr; the other, with dwarf stem and
round seed, ttRR – and postulated that the constitution of the
F_1 plants must be TtRr.

The segregation of the two factors and their recombination
is illustrated in Fig. 16, using the same scheme as in the previous figure.

Mendel expected that the F_1 plants would produce four
types of gametes, and that self-pollination would yield 16
classes. In the second generation, however, he found only four
types of plants:

(a) tall with round seeds, a class like the F_1 plants;
(b) tall with wrinkled seeds, like one of the original parents;
(c) dwarf with round seeds, like the other parent;
(d) dwarf with wrinkled seeds, a *new class* of plants.

The proportion of these types was 9:3:3:1. When Mendel
considered each character separately, he found that the plants
displaying the dominant characters were not uniform; by
self-pollination they produced plants showing dominant and
recessive characters. The ratio for tall/dwarf was 3:1, for
round/wrinkled it was also 3:1.

These results convinced Mendel that his first principle,
according to which the factors of the parental characters
segregate in the offspring, is valid for all characters in which
the parents differ, and, furthermore, that the separation and
recombination of the factors, and consequently the various
characters they influence, are independent of each other. This
is the second law of Mendel.

The number of different characters in the parents determine
the number of possible combinations of the different gametes
produced by the offspring. Thus, when parents differ in one
character only, two kinds of gametes are formed and the
number of possible combinations of the gametes is four; in the
case of two characters, four kinds of gametes are produced
and 16 combinations are possible. When the parents differ in
three characters, the number of combinations possible is 64,
because eight different gametes are produced. In a cross in

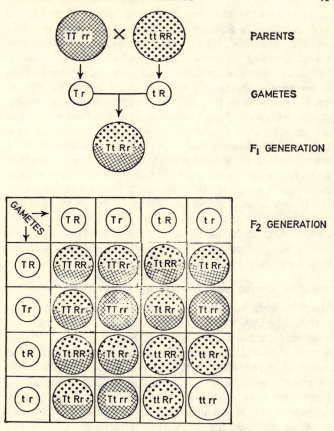

Fig. 16. *Mendel's second law, illustrated in the cross between parents differing in two characters: tall stem (T), wrinkled seed (r), and short stem (t), round seed (R).*

which the parents differ in 10 characters, 1024 types of gametes can be formed; consequently, the number of possible combinations of these characters is 1 048 576.

The Mendelian principles which govern heredity spotlight the origin of the great diversity which exists amongst the members of a species – including our own! Mendel claimed that it is possible 'to determine the number of different forms with certainty in separate generations and to ascertain their statistical relations'. He explained not only the mechanism of heredity, but at the same time threw light on the nature of variation. His contemporaries failed to realise the tremendous importance of the experiments and of the principles Mendel deduced from them. He lived another 19 years after publishing his *Experiments in Plant Hybridisation*, and turned away from experimental work when he became Prelate of the monastery a few years later. Mendel died in 1884. The announcement of his death, drafted by Mendel himself, referred to the numerous social distinctions he received but failed to mention his interest in scientific work. H. Iltis, Mendel's biographer, wrote, 'a kindly and beloved priest rather than a Titan of thought was praised and laid away' on 6 January 1884. Even some biologists of today are inclined to think of Mendel as though he had been a visitor from outer space whose brief transit through European Science was unobserved at the time.

THE CHROMOSOMAL BASIS OF MENDELIAN HEREDITY

Mendel's work and ideas lay forgotten until the turn of the century. The Dutch botanist H. de Vries reported the results of breeding experiments on a large number of plants and referred to similar findings by Mendel. Within a few weeks two more reports were published on the same subject, one in Germany the other in Austria, both mentioning Mendel's experiments. Though his work was rediscovered and proved, opposition to the acceptance of the universal validity of Mendel's interpretation persisted for many years afterwards. One of the reasons for scepticism was the fact that the results of some breeding tests could not be interpreted according to Mendelian principles. To many scientists these principles appeared to be too theoretical, his factors too abstract entities.

The most powerful support for Mendelian heredity came from the cytologist S. Sutton, who recognised that the segregation of chromosomes during gamete formation paralleled the behaviour of Mendel's postulated abstract 'factors'. Sutton wrote in one of his papers published in 1904: 'I call attention to the probability that the association of paternal and maternal chromosomes in pairs and their subsequent separation during the reducing division may constitute the physical basis of the Mendelian law and heredity.'

Sutton realised that the position of chromosome pairs on the equatorial plate is entirely a matter of chance, hence a large number of different combinations of maternal and paternal chromosomes are possible in the mature gametes. Fig. 17 illustrates the parallelism, the segregation and assort-

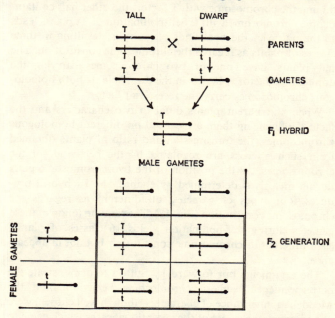

Fig. 17. *Diagram illustrating the chromosomal basis of Mendel's first law.*

ment of the Mendelian 'factors' for tall and dwarf stems of the garden pea as interpreted on the basis of chromosome behaviour.

According to this interpretation the homologous chromosomes are the bearers of the factors T and t. In the parents, both homologous chromosomes carry the same factor: in the tall plant T, in the dwarf pea t. During meiosis these chromosomes pair, and when they segregate only *one kind* of gamete is produced by each parent: all gametes carry a chromosome with T in the tall parent or with t in the dwarf parent. The union of the parental gametes results in hybrid plants (Tt) in which one member of the homologous chromosome pair carries T and the other member t. Segregation of these chromosomes will produce *two kinds* of gametes, half of them containing the chromosome with T factor, the other half containing the chromosome with t. Self-pollination of Tt plants leads to the union of the two kinds of gametes, resulting in three classes of plants as regards the chromosome constitution. The tall plants have one or two chromosomes carrying the dominant T factor, whereas in the dwarf plants both homologous chromosomes carry the recessive t factor.

When the parent plants differ in two characters and the factors influencing them are carried on different homologous chromosomes, the transmission and ratio of plants obtained from such a cross are regulated by the behaviour of the chromosomes. As the position of the two chromosome pairs during meiosis is determined by chance, the F_1 hybrid produces four types of gametes, all different as regards the chromosome constitution (Fig. 18). The random union of these gametes during self-pollination yields 16 classes of plants, each different in chromosome constitution but not in appearance.

The arguments put forward by Sutton to demonstrate the correspondence between chromosome behaviour and the Mendelian inheritance of characters, though well chosen, were not convincing because of the exceptional cases which came to light in breeding experiments. The evidence which could have shown that the laws of Mendel are dictated by the chromosomes was lacking for many years to come. The definite proof that the chromosomes are the vehicle of the Mendelian factors, and, furthermore, that only on this basis can the apparent exceptions to Mendelian heredity be explained, was provided by the geneticists of the succeeding decade. The vision of

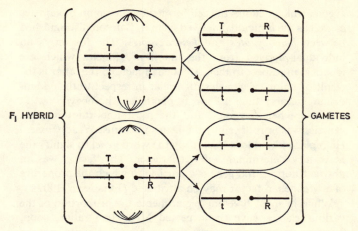

Fig. 18. *Diagram illustrating the chromosomal basis of Mendel's second law; the type of segregation of the two pairs of homologous chromosomes in F_1 hybrids depends on their arrangements at metaphase.*

Sutton that 'the chromosomes represent a group of associated hereditary units' became true with the discoveries of T. H. Morgan and his co-workers at Columbia University, New York (see Appendix II).

THE GENETIC STRUCTURE OF CHROMOSOMES

The rediscovery of Mendel's work and the theoretical principles postulated by him, stimulated botanists and zoologists to test their validity. In England, W. Bateson was the leading experimentalist who put to test the Mendelian interpretation of heredity in animals. He crossed different varieties of rabbits and poultry, and his results confirmed the findings of Mendel. Bateson coined new technical terms to indicate more precisely the various phenomena encountered in the breeding tests. To him we owe the name 'genetics', the study of the mechanism of heredity. Bateson introduced the term *allele*, indicating the alternative character, e.g. 'tall' stem is an allele of 'short' stem, 'round' seed is allele of 'wrinkled' seed. Accepting the term *zygote*, which denotes the cell formed by the union of gametes as well as the individual derived from it, Bateson distinguished between *homozygotes* and *heterozygotes*. The former is an individual derived from the union of gametes which are identical in respect to their Mendelian factors, the latter is the result of union of gametes dissimilar in respect to their Mendelian factors; thus TT or tt plants are homozygotes, Tt plants are heterozygotes. But the most important term in genetics was introduced by the Danish botanist W. Johanssen. He replaced Mendel's 'factor' by the word *gene*, to signify the hereditary determinant of a character. The 'factor' was an abstract notion, the gene is a particle to which the properties of a Mendelian factor may be attributed (Johanssen, 1909).

While in most breeding experiments the proportion of the various classes gave the expected Mendelian ratios, soon, however, observations were reported which could not be explained on Mendel's principles. Such findings were used as arguments against Mendel. R. C. Punnett, the pupil of Bateson, observed that in crossing varieties of sweet peas which differed in two characters, (a) the colour of the flower and (b) the shape of the pollen, the ratio of the four classes obtained in the second generation deviated very much from the 9:3:3:1 ratio; the homozygotes, i.e. the plants showing the two dominant and the two recessive characters were much more numerous than was expected, indicating that their factors failed to segregate. In view of these results, Punnett came to the conclusion that the Mendelian factors of the two characters must be in some manner 'coupled', or linked together, and therefore could not segregate in the hybrid independently into separate gametes. Many similar deviations from the Mendelian ratios were observed, which, however, could all be explained by assuming that the hereditary determinants of the characters – Mendel's factors or Johanssen's genes – are linked together.

The linkage of characters has been demonstrated by Morgan and his pupils on a very impressive scale in Drosophila, the 'black-bellied dew lover'. It is a small insect and a very suitable organism to make breeding tests with, as its life cycle is short (15–20 days), it is easy to breed, and one mating produces several hundred offspring. Within a year of breeding the fruit fly, Morgan's pupils found many specimens showing new characters, e.g. white eye-colour, short bristles, truncated wing, dumpy body shape, etc. These characters were extensively used in genetic experiments; their method of inheritance was studied, and their relationship to each other was clarified. According to the results obtained in the second generation flies, Morgan could arrange the various characters into four 'linkage groups'. Some of the characters of the various groups are given in Table 4.

Table 4. *Mutants in Drosophila.*

Group 1	Group 2	Group 3	Group 4
Bar (eye-shape)	Black (body-colour)	Beaded (wing)	Bent (wing)
Cherry (eye-colour)	Blistered (wing)	Claret (eye-colour)	Eyeless (eye)
Eosin (eye-colour)	Purple (eye-colour)	Dwarf (body)	
Forked (spine)	Truncate (wing)	Deformed (eye)	
Miniature (wing)	Vestigial (wing)	Peach (eye-colour)	
Notch (venation)		Sepia (eye-colour)	
Vermilion (eye)			
Yellow (body-colour)			

The most remarkable fact was, however, the close correspondence between the number of the linkage groups and the number of chromosome pairs, i.e. the haploid number. In Drosophila there are eight chromosomes which are arranged into four pairs, and Morgan could establish only four linkage groups from the breeding tests. Other scientists discovered linkage of characters in the sweet pea, maize, mice and other organisms all confirming Morgan's observation that the number of linkage groups in a species is the same as the number of chromosome pairs.

It was, however, soon found that linkage between two characters is not permanent, since individuals always turned up in the experiments which had only one of the characters which were known to be linked. How could it happen that the genes of these characters segregated during gamete formation? To explain this phenomenon, Morgan turned to the 'chiasma-type theory' put forward in 1909 by Janssens. According to this theory, the chiasma which is formed during meiosis represents an exchange of corresponding parts of chromatids of homologous chromosomes. Morgan argued that this is a process most suitable to separate linked genes from each other and to transfer one to the homologous partner chromosome. Morgan looked upon the chiasma as the cytological evidence of the 'crossing-over' of genes (1913). Fig. 19 illustrates this process

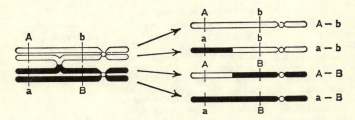

Fig. 19. *Chiasma formation between homologous chromosome showing crossing-over between the genes* A *and* B.

and shows the new arrangement of genes due to chiasma formation between the paired homologous chromosomes. The chance to form chiasma between any two given points in the same chromosome increases with the distance between these points. The frequency of crossing-over between two genes which are located on the same chromosomes indicates the distance between them; low frequency suggests that the two genes are near to each other, high numbers indicate a larger distance. The occurrence of crossing-over between linked genes made possible the construction of chromosome 'maps' in which the genes are placed into definite positions along the chromosomes.

The excellent work of the Morgan school established firmly the fact that the genes, the 'units of heredity', are arranged in *linear order* on the chromosomes, each having a fixed position in relation to the other genes. Sutton only demonstrated the likelihood that the chromosomes are the bearers of Mendelian factors, the Morgan school proved this beyond doubt. Furthermore, the impressive results of the Drosophila experiments provided an explanation for the deviations from the expected Mendelian ratios. The 'exceptional class' occurred only in those breeding tests in which characters belonging to the same linkage groups had been used.

The geneticists of today realise how fortunate Mendel was when he chose the garden pea for his experiments. We know now that the genes of the different characters he studied are not linked, they are all located in different chromosomes. If it had been otherwise, the new combination of the genes due to crossing-over could have given him variable and unpredictable numerical results which would have prevented Mendel formulating his 'laws'.

LINKAGE OF GENES WITH SEX

One of the most convincing pieces of evidence that chromosomes are the physical basis of heredity was the identification of the chromosome in which the gene of a particular character is located. The character was the white eye-colour of Drosophila, discovered in 1908. In the eyes of such flies, the pigment responsible for the red eye-colour of the 'normal', or wild type, is completely absent.

Morgan crossed white-eyed male Drosophila with wild-type females with red eyes, and from the mating obtained flies all having red eyes, which indicated that red eye-colour is dominant and the white is recessive. On crossing females and males of the F_1 hybrid, Morgan expected, according to the Mendelian law, three times more red than white eye-coloured flies, but he obtained many more red than white. Furthermore, he also noticed that none of the female flies had white eyes, while half of the males had. Such a distribution of the red and white eye-colours amongst the flies of the second generation in respect to sex, could not be accounted for by pure coincidence. To clarify the cause underlying this unexpected finding, Morgan made a reciprocal crossing, by mating white-eyed females with red-eyed males. The result of this mating was even more unexpected than the previous one; Morgan found that all the male flies had white eyes and the females had red eyes, i.e. the inheritance of white eye-colour followed a criss-cross scheme – the mother's character was transmitted to all her sons, while the father's to all his daughters.

To explain the unexpected segregation, Morgan postulated that the gene of red eye-colour and its alternative, or allele, the gene of white eye-colour, are located on the sex chromosome, which was proved to be the X chromosome since the other sex chromosome is present only in the males. The Drosophila experiments showed also that the Y chromosome does not carry the alleles of genes located in the X chromosome, and therefore all the recessive genes can express themselves in spite of the fact that they are present in the male flies as single units (hemizygous). To express themselves in the females, both X chromosomes must carry the recessive gene (homo-zygous). The inheritance of the red and white eye-colours is illustrated in Fig. 20 according to the interpretation by Morgan.

Morgan's breeding results and similar findings of other investigators during the following years revealed the criteria by which a character can be considered to be sex-linked. The two most important are: (a) that the number of individuals with such a character is much higher in the male sex than in the female sex and (b) that it is never transmitted from the male parent to the sons.

A good example of a sex-linked *recessive* trait in man is red–green colour-blindness. This condition is fairly widespread, but fortunately the red and green traffic lights also differ in brightness, and the motorist who is colour-blind can recognise the difference between 'stop' and 'go'. Mothers with normal eyesight can be 'carriers' of the gene for colour-blindness (the gene being present only in one of their X chromosomes) and in this case they can have sons who are colour-blind. The 'car-rier' becomes very important if the recessive gene she carries determines a serious condition such as haemophilia, or bleeding disease, known since ancient times. There is a refer-ence in the Talmud (A.D. 150) to the 'uncontrollable bleeding'

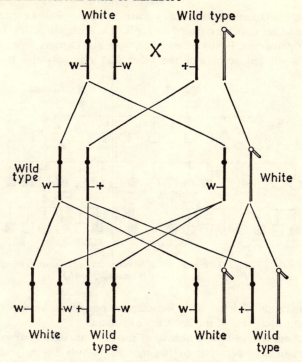

Fig. 20. *Sex linkage in* Drosophila; *both X chromosomes of the female carry the gene* w *for white eye-colour; the X of the male carries the normal* (+) *wild type allele.* (*X chromosome is black.*)

causing the death of circumcised boys. In this disease the blood from a wound fails to clot as there is a deficiency of a particular protein in the serum. Haemophiliacs lose large amounts of blood from the smallest wound, and even minor operations such as extraction of a tooth can be fatal for them. In families in which the gene for haemophilia is transmitted, no apparently normal woman can feel sure that she is not a 'carrier'. Haemophilia has become widely known since its occurrence in the royal families of Europe, including ours. The transmission of this fatal condition in the various royal families is shown in

Fig. 21. Queen Victoria was a 'carrier' of the gene. Leopold, one of her sons, died from haemophilia at the age of 31. Two of her daughters, Beatrice and Alice, were also carriers; one had two affected sons, and the other had one son and three

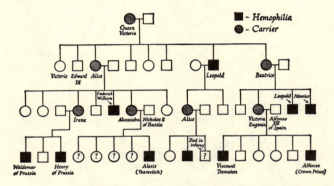

Fig. 21. *Inheritance of haemophilia in the royal families of Europe. (After A. M. Winchester, 1964.)*

grandsons afflicted with the disease, one of whom was the Tsarevitch, son of the last Czar of Russia.

Another sex-linked disease of man is muscular dystrophy (progressive paralysis of the muscles) which affects young boys, becoming apparent when the child starts to walk. The condition rapidly progresses, and at about the age of 10 the child's legs become useless, he is confined to an invalid chair and dies a few years later. As the boy dies in his early teens, it is totally unlikely that he will father any children. This fatal, sex-linked disease can therefore exist only through unaffected carriers! Investigation is going on at present to find some method by which carriers of this condition can be recognised. This is the first step towards eliminating the disease.

Recently a disease, neonatal jaundice due to the deficiency of the enzyme G6PD (Glucose-6-phosphate dehydrogenase), was found to be caused by a recessive gene situated on the X chromosome. The female heterozygotes (carriers) of this metabolic disorder can be identified by taking a sample of blood and measuring the level of the enzyme G6PD; this is much lower in the carriers than in the non-carriers.

The most clear-cut example of sex-linked *dominant* inheritance is provided by the blood group Xg, discovered in 1962. A female parent homozygous for Xg, will produce daughters and sons all belonging to the mother's blood group, Xg, irrespective of what the father's blood group was. On the other hand, the Xg gene of the father is never transmitted to his sons.

The four traits have been found in families in various combinations, making it possible to obtain crossing-over data and to place them in certain positions. Fig. 22 shows the location

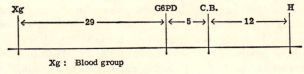

Xg : Blood group

G6PD : Neonatal jaundice

C.B. : Colour blindness

H : Haemophilia

Fig. 22. *The position of genes in the human X chromosome.*

of the four genes relative to each other in the X chromosome of man.

It has been already stated that the genes of the X chromosome have no corresponding alleles in the Y chromosome; it seems, and it is supported by various evidence, that the genes in the Y are primarily concerned with sex determination. In man, there is at present only one well-substantiated Y-linked character – 'hairy pinna of the ear' – which is exclusively passed down on the male line. Though the sex of the new individual is determined at the moment of fertilisation, the decisive part in the development of the sexual characteristics is played by the sex hormones secreted by the ovary and testes in vertebrate animals. If the testes are removed from a 'pre-adolescent' boy, he will fail to develop the features characteristic of the male sex; similarly, the removal of the ovaries from young females arrests the development of female characteristics. The specific genes of the X and Y chromosomes are believed to control the type of hormones to be produced in the developing organism.*

Anomalies in the constitution of the sex chromosomes can occur, and because of the hormonal disturbance which follows, an abnormal sexual state is produced in the individual concerned. The hormonal function may be readjusted by operative intervention, but for this to be successful it is important to determine the constitution of the sex chromosome, i.e. the 'genetic sex' of the person. Important progress was made in this respect when in 1949 Murray Barr discovered the '*sex chromatin*', a mass of chromatin present in the interphase nucleus of most cells in females, which is only very rarely seen in males. The sex chromatin, often called the 'Barr-body', can easily be recognised in the epithelial cells of oral mucosa, and in the white blood cells in which it appears as a 'drumstick'. It is now believed that the sex chromatin is one of the X chromosomes in the female cell in a condensed state. The rule is established that the number of sex chromatins is one less than the number of Xes. In normal males with XY sex chromosomes, it is absent; in an abnormal female with XXX constitution, the number of sex chromatins is two.

Recently, Dr Mary Lyon at Harwell suggested that the genes in the chromosome which forms the sex chromatin are inactivated. Lyon's hypothesis is based on the behaviour of coat colour in mice. She found mottled female mice which were heterozygous for a gene determining a dominant coat colour. The mottled fur was due to the appearance of the recessive coat colour, the gene of which is present in one of the X chromosomes. Lyon attributed the appearance of the recessive coat colour to the inactivation of the dominant gene during embryonic development. According to her view, the size of the patches showing the recessive colour indicates when the inactivation occurred in the embryo.

* The role of sex chromosomes and hormones in sexual differentiation has been surveyed recently by R. J. Harrison in *Reproduction and Man* (C.S.P.3). Oliver & Boyd, 1967.

In discussing the sex chromosomes and their genes, attention must be drawn to the difference between the sex-linked traits and autosomal characters. The latter are determined by genes which are always present in pairs. This, however, does not hold for the X-linked genes; they are present in pairs in females (XX), but singly in males, yet their effects are identical. It is found that green and red colour-blindness of the 'hemizygous' male, for instance, is the same as in the homozygous female. It is not known how, but it seems that in the male the single X compensates for the dose-difference. The hypothesis of Lyon takes this phenomenon into consideration.

Before closing our discussion on the genetic aspect of the sex chromosomes, we should mention the unequal ratio observed between males and females in man. As the male sex produces X and Y chromosomes carrying gametes in equal proportions, accordingly the sex ratio expected would be 1:1 between the two sexes. However, this is not the case. The ratio is 106:100 for boys and girls born in the United States. The deviation cannot be attributed to the fact that more female babies die in the womb during pregnancy than boys. Studies indicate that the ratio is already altered in the very early human embryos, which suggests that the Y-carrying sperm has some advantage over the sperm carrying the X chromosome. Investigation is in progress in several laboratories to identify the property which could give such an advantage; when this is known it may be possible to influence sex determination. Economically it would be very profitable to produce more females than males in certain domestic animals, or vice versa. If such methods succeed, no doubt they will be adapted for man. Instances have also been reported in which the sex ratio is influenced by genes. Several family pedigrees are on record in which there is a great preponderance of females through several generations. It is also known that sex can influence the manifestation of certain inherited traits, e.g. gout is 20 times more frequent in males than in females; on the other hand, diabetes is more frequent in females. At present we have no explanation for this phenomenon.

3. Genes in Action

The view that the chromosomes are aggregates of genes, each having a place which is strictly fixed in linear order, was a very useful concept, helping the geneticists to understand the mechanism of Mendelian heredity on a material basis and to explain apparent inconsistencies found in breeding experiments. The evidence was convincing that inheritance is based on pairs of particular units, the genes. How many such units are required to determine a particular character or trait? How do genes regulate the complex chemical reactions, the end product of which is a cell differentiated to fulfil a specific function? How can the concept of the gene, as was formulated by Morgan and by the followers of classical genetics, be fitted into our present-day knowledge of the DNA? These are some of the problems to be discussed in this chapter.

INTERACTION AND CUMULATIVE EFFECTS OF GENES

The breeding experiments with plants and animals produced many results that threw more light on the operation of Mendelian heredity. It was observed that in certain crosses the F_1 hybrid did not show the dominant character, but was either intermediate or exhibited an entirely new characteristic. Thus when a red flower snapdragon was crossed to a white variety, the hybrid had pink flowers; when a red bull is mated to a white cow, the offspring are roan in colour, i.e. intermediate between the two parents. The Andalusian, a domestic fowl, has feathers of a steel-blue colour produced when a white variety and a black variety are crossed. These observations of the early geneticists indicated that the chain of events initiated by the genes which control the production of pigments responsible for the colour varieties must have interacted in some manner during development. In these instances the interaction occurs between alleles, i.e. genes which occupy corresponding loci in homologous chromosomes.

When analysing the genetic basis of the various coat colours in rabbit or the shapes of the comb in poultry, in order to explain the breeding results, W. Bateson and R. C. Punnett had to postulate that these characters were influenced or controlled by several factors, in some cases by two, in others by three genes. They also discovered that when the genes were combined, new characters appeared in the first generation hybrid. From crossing two varieties of poultry, one with a rose-comb and the other with a pea-comb, Bateson obtained birds with walnut-combs; a new form.

A very interesting example of gene interaction is provided by the coat colour of mice, which is controlled by two genes, A and B, and their recessive alleles, a and b. The combination of these genes produces the wild-type agouti (AABB), black (aaBB), cinnamon (AAbb) and chocolate (aabb). The cross of black with cinnamon yields agouti mice; when these agoutis are crossed, all four kinds of coat colour appear in the ratio of 9 agouti : 3 cinnamon : 3 black : 1 chocolate.

In Drosophila there are 15 genes, which on acting together produce the red eye-colour of the wild-type fly. Homozygous recessive alleles of any of these genes alter the red eye-colour. When two or more such alleles are present, the colour of the eye is still further modified.

In all instances the genes which interact to influence the same character occupy separate positions in the chromosomes; some may be located on the same chromosome, while others may be widely distributed on several non-homologous chromosomes, i.e. belonging to different linkage groups. Such genes whose combined action affects one particular character are known as *multiple genes*, or *polygenes*, each of which have only one other alternative form, or allele.

Many instances are known in plants and animals in which the same character is controlled by several genes. In man, the disease of muscles (muscular dystrophy) is such a condition, where three genes have been identified as being responsible: one is a sex-linked recessive gene already discussed, the second is an autosomal recessive, and the third is an autosomal dominant gene.

There are at least four genes responsible for the colour of our skin; they control in some manner the amount of melanin pigment deposited in the skin. The children of European and Negro marriages – the mulattos – have dark skin nearer in colour to that of the Negro parent. When two mulattos marry, the colour of the children may range from nearly white to black. As there are four genes segregating, we can expect from 256 such mixed marriages one completely white or black child.

Height or size are other characters which are determined by polygenes. Their single effects are small and cannot be observed separately, but the great variation seen in heights of large groups of individuals is the result of the variable combination of these genes. Measurements of height in population show a continuous gradation, and even close relatives vary in size from their parents as well as amongst themselves. One of the first geneticists to study the genetic basis of size was Punnett, who crossed the small Sebright Bantam fowl with the large Golden Hamburg and in the second generation obtained birds some of which were larger and some smaller than the grandparents. The extreme types as regards size were the result of a particular combination of the multiple genes.

Other examples of such characters are life-span, degree of resistance to disease, age of onset of a disease, rate of heart beat, length of fingers, arterial blood pressure, rate of function of thyroid gland, and many other inherited traits. The concept that polygenes are the basis of quantitative characters provides an insight into the causes of variability seen in many plants and animals; the aim of modern genetics is to separate the individual components of the genes from their cumulative effect. By using the number of hairs in certain abdominal segments of the fruit fly, K. Mather and B. J. Harrison have shown that the difference in variation observed in two strains was due to polygenes and that the contribution of the genes, localised in the three major chromosomes, was different. They demonstrated that the basis of continuous variation is the simultaneous operation of a number of genes. Although they cannot be analysed by the Mendelian method, the individual genes, components of the polygenic system, are inherited in accordance with the Mendelian principles.

SUBGENES: THE MULTIPLE ALLELES

In the instances we have just discussed, the genes affect the same character although they occupy different loci in the chromosomes. It has also been found that one gene can have a whole series of alternatives, each affecting the same character to a different degree. The significance of this phenomenon is in the fact that the 'alternatives' are all within the confine of the same gene, i.e. the gene is in some manner subdivided into alleles. The first such example was provided by the eye-colour of Drosophila studied by Morgan and his school. They found that when a male fly with 'eosin' coloured eyes was crossed with a female having 'white' eyes, the sons all had white eyes, whilst the daughters had eyes of a colour between eosin and white. The transmission of the white eye-colour from the mother to her sons indicated that the gene is located in the X chromosome. Breeding tests have also shown that the genes of white and eosin could not be recombined. In view of this finding, Morgan postulated that the two genes must be alleles to each other and must therefore occupy the same locus. Further tests have shown that Morgan's assumption was correct. We now know 14 varieties of the gene which affect eye-colour in Drosophila; these gene varieties are called *multiple alleles*. To discriminate the members in the series, a superscript is added to the same symbol: W = red (normal eye-colour, wild type, dominant); w = white, w^e = eosin, w^a = apricot, w^c = coral, w^i = ivory, all recessives, but they produce intermediate eye-colours in the hybrid.

In man, the blood groups are determined by multiple alleles. The blood groups, discovered in 1901 by K. Landsteiner, and distinguished by the *antigens*, are specific proteins located on the surface of the red blood cells. They are identified by means of the *antibodies*, another kind of protein, present in the serum of the blood. In certain combinations the antigens and antibodies link together, and the aggregates of red blood cells form clots which can cause the death of the individual. At present, 14 blood-group systems have been discovered in man, and each system is controlled by different genes which form a series of alleles. Here we are going to discuss only two: ABO and Rh blood groups.

In the ABO blood group, genes A and B are co-dominant; when both are present, the red blood cells carry antigen-A and antigen-B. Gene O is recessive; the red blood cells of a person whose blood group is O have no antigens. The A, B and O genes occupy the same locus on the chromosome; in any one individual, therefore, only two genes can be present. The following four blood groups are possible: O (each homologous chromosome carries the recessive genes O/O); A (the gene constitution is A/A or A/O); B (the gene constitution is B/B or B/O); and AB (one chromosome carries gene A, the other gene B). A and B genes have two functions: they determine the specificity of the antigen on the red blood cells and control the production of antibodies in the serum. A gene produces anti-B, B gene produces anti-A antibodies; anti-B protein agglutinates the red blood cells of a person who belongs to B blood group and vice versa, anti-A agglutinates the red blood cells of group A. Individuals of O blood group have no antigen on the red blood cells; they have, on the other hand, antibodies against the red blood cells of A and B groups. The co-dominant AB genes together produce antigen A and B but not antibodies. The antibodies of A, B and O alleles are already present in the foetus, therefore they are referred to as 'natural antibodies' to distinguish them from those produced only when a person comes into contact with foreign proteins or antigens. The reactions of the red blood cells of A, B, AB, and O individuals to the various antibodies are shown in Table 5.

Blood groups are man's most useful stamp of identity. The mode of inheritance of the genes responsible for them is simple. By knowing the blood groups of parents, the children's possible blood group can be predicted and, vice versa, the blood group of children can indicate to what group their

Table 5. *The properties of blood groups.*

Blood group	Recipient Antibodies in serum	Blood group of donor			
		O	A	B	AB
O	anti-A, anti-B	−	+	+	+
A	anti-B	−	−	+	+
B	anti-A	−	+	−	+
AB	neither	−	−	−	−

+ = agglutination − = no agglutination

parents belong. Table 6 shows the different blood-group types of children who could be born to parents belonging to a particular ABO blood group.

Table 6. *Inheritance of blood groups.*

Parental blood type	Possible blood types of children
O × A	O, A
O × B	O, B
O × AB	A, B
A × A	O, A
A × B	O, A, B, AB
A × AB	A, B, AB
B × B	O, B
B × AB	A, B, AB
AB × AB	A, B, AB

The blood group is valuable evidence in cases where there is a question of true parentage. Although paternity can never be proved with absolute certainty, it can always be disproved. A child of B blood group cannot have parents whose blood groups are O and A; a man of O group cannot be the father of an AB child. According to the rule of heredity, a man cannot be the father if his and the child's mother's blood groups differ from the blood group of the child. Similarly, an O child cannot claim a man with AB glood group to be his father, since the child must have one of the dominant genes and its antigen which the putative father has.

Blood groups are also extensively used to determine whether twins are identical or not, and they prove to be most useful in clinical practice when blood transfusion is necessary.

The Rhesus (Rh) blood-group system was discovered in 1940 when red blood cells of the *rhesus* monkey were injected into rabbits. The antibodies produced in rabbits as a result of the injection agglutinated the red cells of the rhesus. It was also found that when rabbit serum with anti-Rh antibodies is mixed with human red blood cells, the red blood cells agglutinated in some cases. The individuals whose red cells are agglutinated are Rh-positive (Rh+) because they have the specific Rh-antigen on the surface of their red blood cells; others, whose blood cells do not react, lack this antigen and are called Rh-negative (Rh−).

This blood group has great clinical importance due to a fatal disease in the newborn called erythroblastosis foetalis. The condition is due to incompatibility between the blood of the foetus and that of the mother, the foetus being Rh+ and the mother Rh−. Towards the end of pregnancy or during labour, the blood of the Rh+ baby may enter into the mother's blood circulation through the placenta, and the Rh antigen on the baby's red cells induces the mother's immunological defences to produce antibodies against it. Normally, the first baby is unaffected, but the Rh antibodies produced in the mother by the first child's blood cells remain in her circulation and prepare a death-trap for later children. The mother's antibodies enter into the Rh+ baby and destroy the red blood cells, causing severe anaemia, jaundice and often death.

The 'Rh' gene is inherited as a simple dominant; it differs from the A or B genes of ABO blood group in that it does not produce anti-Rh antibodies in the serum of Rh-positive people. An Rh+ person should never be a donor of blood for an Rh− individual. In the first instance the transfusion may not be fatal because the transfused red-cells with their Rh antigen would be replaced before the Rh− person produced sufficient antibodies against them, but agglutination of Rh+ blood cells will occur at the second transfusion or at the second pregnancy of an Rh+ baby.

In Britain 12 per cent of all marriages are between an Rh+ husband and Rh— wife, and every year about 300 babies die from erythroblastosis. During the last few years much research has been done to find methods which could prevent the development of this fatal condition. One method is the replacement of the infant's Rh+ blood cells with Rh— cells; extensive blood transfusions can replace many of the damaged red blood cells and save the child during the critical days immediately before or after birth. Some babies may, however, need several intra-uterine transfusions, and each is a risky operation. Recently doctors in Liverpool introduced a new measure. They argued that the Rh+ cells which entered the mother from the baby at birth could be destroyed by anti-Rh serum containing antibodies against them, if it were injected immediately after the birth. This method is used now on an increasing scale, and measures are already under way to provide adequate supplies of the serum with anti-Rh antibodies to treat mothers who could give birth to a second Rh+ child.

Studies of the Rh blood-group system revealed several kinds of antigens (C, D and E), but their genetic basis is still a matter of debate. Some geneticists argue that the Rh gene and its three alleles occupy a single locus in the chromosome. Others believe that the antigens are determined by three distinct genes, C, D and E, which occupy loci close together in the chromosome and behave like multiple alleles. In the Rh system the 'subgene' responsible for the D antigen is the most important.

Transferrin (Tf) is another example of multiple allelism in man. It is a special type of protein present in the blood plasma and has an important role in binding and transporting iron. We know about 18 varieties of transferrin identified by electrophoresis, a process based on the different migration rates of ions in an electric field. The variant forms of transferrin are inherited as simple co-dominant Mendelian traits reflecting the action of a series of alleles at one locus like the alleles of blood groups. It is of some interest to note that one of the variants, Tf-D, shows a high frequency amongst African Negroes, Australian Aborigines and Melanesians. The curious distribution of this protein raises important problems in respect of human evolution. Did the Tf-D variant originate before these races separated? Did it arise independently in the different populations? Did it spread by migration? These are interesting and important questions, and studies are at present in progress to find the answers.

The blood-group systems were the first illustration of multiple allelism in man. Many traits are now known, the inheritance of which indicates that they are controlled by multiple alleles. The study of such traits is important because they provide a good example of *direct* control of particular characters by genes.

THE GENETIC BASIS OF INDIVIDUALITY

It has been mentioned that when the red blood cells of an Rh+ baby enter the Rh— mother, they induce a reaction; this consists of the production of antibodies specifically directed against the baby's red blood cells, resulting in their agglutination. The intruders are thus rendered harmless and are removed from the mother's system by scavenger cells. This reaction is referred to as the immune response; it is triggered off by antigens, the protein molecules sited on the surface of the foreign cells. The antigens of the red blood cells are mucopolysaccharides, those of tissue cells are lipoproteins. The antigens are recognised by particular cells, members of the defence mechanism of the body. The specificity of the antigens is controlled by genes, one gene determining one antigen. The antibodies are serum proteins of the gamma globulin class, having the power to pair with two antigen molecules. The body or, to be more correct, the particular cells in the body can synthesise an apparently endless variety of specific antibodies when challenged by specific antigens of a foreign organism (bacteria or cells). These are antigens which are 'species specific' and distinguish one species from another; for instance, by the help of these antigens we can easily find out whether the blood in the gut of the mosquito is that of a man or a cow.

The location of antigens on the surface of cells can be

revealed by the use of fluorescent dyes. The dye conjugates with the antibody and the fluorescence which shows up under ultraviolet light indicates the sites attacked by the antibodies. Similarly, the same technique can be applied to reveal the antigenic sites on cells.

The intrusion of bacteria, virus or cells into an organism sets into motion the immune mechanism, which in most cases controls, kills or rejects the intruders and then remains as an effective protection against a second challenge from the same organism, thereby establishing immunity. Tissues and organs transplanted between genetically unrelated individuals of the same species are called *homografts*; they do not normally survive for longer than a week or two. On the other hand, grafts between genetically identical individuals (e.g. identical twins, mice of the same inbred strains) are accepted; these are called *isografts*. Tissue grafts donated by an animal to itself are most favoured; these are the *autografts* used in plastic surgery. The rejection of homografts indicates that donor and recipient are incompatible due to genetic differences between them. The differences are expressed by the presence of 'transplantation antigens', which are elaborated by nucleated cells.

The genetic basis of tissue transplantation has been clarified from studies of mice. The transplantation of skin or other tissues between mice belonging to different inbred strains produced by brother–sister matings through many generations, showed that the antigenic substances responsible for provoking immunological response are controlled by genes. In mice, so far 15 such genes have been identified, each occupying a separate locus in different chromosomes. One such gene, designated as H-2, is the most investigated histocompatibility gene. It was recognised in the early 1930s by Dr J. Gorer at Guy's Hospital, London. The H-2 gene has at least 18 alleles, each determining different antigens, which already appear in early foetal life. The transplantation antigens, like the red cell antigens, are located at or near the surface of tissue cells. How incompatibility operates in transplantation is illustrated in Fig. 23.

The various responses when skin grafts are exchanged between two mice, belonging to different strains, and between their offspring (F₁ hybrid) are indicated. Assuming that the

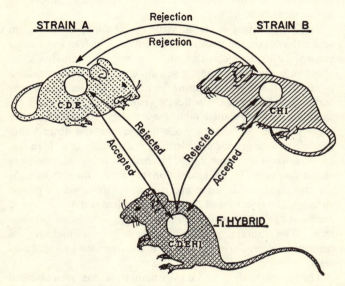

Fig. 23. *The fate of skin grafts exchanged between parents and F₁ hybrid differing in transplantation antigens.*

antigenic constitution of the parental strains is CDE and CHI respectively, out of the three antigens only C is common to both. By mating the two parents, the F₁ hybrid will have the histocompatibility genes and transplantation antigens of both parents; it can therefore accept parental skin grafts. The fate of the F₁ hybrid's skin on the parents, however, is quite different; it is rejected by both parents because the A-parent reacts against the HI antigens and the B-parent against the DE antigens; these antigens are present in the hybrid but absent in the respective parents.

In the rejection of tissue or organ grafts, antibodies circulating in the blood play very little if any part at all. The rejection of the homograft is mediated by particular cells, the lympho-cytes, which are produced in certain sites, e.g. lymph nodes, spleen, etc. These cells have the ability to recognise the for-eign nature of antigens. It has been found that the antigens of the grafted tissue diffuse into the lymph and reach the sites where the lymphocytes are. The cells become 'activated', migrate towards the graft, infiltrate into the tissue and, by a process not yet understood, destroy it. It is now believed that the immune reaction against the homograft is the chief ob-stacle to clinical organ transplantation, prevening successful replacement of diseased organs such as kidney, liver or lung. It is a tragic paradox that a patient's own defence mechanism frustrates th eefforts of clinicians and surgeons, efforts which are aimed at saving his life.

Incompatibility is absent between identical twins. They can tolerate skin grafts and transplantation of organs between one another. Such twins arise from the fertilisation of the same egg-cell and have identical genes and antigens. The rule of homograft does not apply to identical twins because their genetic constitution is the same. In rare instances the 'homo-graft barrier' can be broken. Such is the case when grafting cornea, bone or blood vessels; this kind of homograft is accepted and survives because of the peculiar nature of these tissues or graft-bed.

In view of the urgent need for 'spare-part surgery' in desperate situations, various methods are under test to cir-cumvent or suppress the reaction of the recipient patient against the homograft. It was found that grafts are better tolerated if the genetic difference between the individual donating the graft and the person receiving it is small. In clinical cases of transplantation, a parent, brother, or sister of the patient is always preferred as the donor since the antigenic difference is less between them than between a patient and unrelated individuals.

The 'Third Report of the Human Kidney Transplant Registry' summarised recently the results on 374 kidney graftings, applying the various methods mentioned above. The report shows that even when the best immunosuppressive method is applied, the survival time of transplanted organs was chiefly determined by the genetic relationship; when close relatives were selected as donors, kidney grafts did survive and function longest.

Recently an investigation has been initiated on a world-wide scale, the aim of which is to identify the transplantation antigens in man. The findings would no doubt greatly facilitate the selection of suitable donors. Temporary suppression of the immune response can be produced by massive doses of irradiation or drugs known as antimetabolites. On the other hand, patients whose immune response is suppressed have a greatly increased risk of infection, and they therefore will require extreme care and attention. The precaution against infection is provided by the 'reverse-barrier' method of nursing, which keeps the patient under aseptic conditions.

During the last two years a new approach has been made towards controlling the immune response. The lymphocytes, cells directly involved in the immune reaction, are injected into rabbit, sheep or horse, and the 'antilymphocyte serum' (ALS) injected into the prospective recipient of the homograft. By this method significant prolongation of homograft survival has been achieved in animals. The method is still in the experimental stage, its applicability to man is yet to be investigated.

Recently it was discovered that in the development of immunological competence of the organism the thymus gland plays an important role. Studies are in progress to throw light on the process by which the role of thymus is exercised in this aspect with the view of controlling the immune response. The aim is very ambitious indeed. The immunological defence mechanism of the organism has developed through millions of years into a highly efficient system. It is based on the specificity of the antigens and on the recognition of their specificity by the body. Recent experiments in which cells of mice and men were 'hybridised', i.e. fused when cultured together *in vitro*, show that the nature of the antigens on the surface of the hybrid cells was determined by the human chromosomes present. This ingenious method revealed that there are many genes controlling the human antigens and that they are widely distributed on the 23 pairs of chromosomes.

At present much effort is being devoted to 'type' the antigens of the white blood cells which are believed to be related to the transplantation antigens. Scientists in the Netherlands found a way to recognise various categories of white blood cells, and so far 12 have been characterised.

When the immunological defences of the recipient are depressed by X-rays or drugs, and the transplanted tissue such as bone marrow contains immunologically competent cells, the graft can react against the host. The syndrome associated with the 'graft versus host' reaction is referred to as runt, or homologous disease, and often terminates in death. Such a syndrome has been observed in children with acute lymphocytic leukaemia, whose diseased bone marrow was destroyed by radiation and who were then injected with bone marrow from healthy donors.

The body's own defence mechanism does not react against its own antigens because the lymphocytes competent to do so become tolerant to them during foetal life and recognise them as 'self'. Antigenic change may occur, however, due for instance to viral infection or to disease. In the latter case, the antigen, which for many years was present but was inaccessible to the cells of the body defence mechanism, is released from the tissue. Against this antigen, an attack would mount, and the antibodies produced could inflict serious damage on the particular tissue harbouring the antigen. Some of the diseases which seem to be due to 'auto-immune' reaction are listed in Table 7.

Transplantation experiments in animals, in which tumours were used, revealed the fact that those produced by chemicals and viruses liberate antigens specific to the tumour but foreign to the tumour-bearing animal. It was found that when very low numbers of tumour cells were transplanted into isologous hosts, tumour development was arrested, indicating that the body's defence system was able to mount a successful attack against the tumour. Spontaneous regression, though very rare, can also occur in human cancer. During the period

Table 7. *Auto-immune diseases.*

Disease	Effect
Lupus erythematosis	Inflammatory disease of the skin, usually on the face
Rheumatoid arthritis	Inflammatory reaction in the joints and cartilage
Hashimoto thyroiditis	Inflammation in the thyroid gland
Myasthenia gravis	Generalised fatigue of muscles
Infantile eczema	Skin lesion
Multiple sclerosis	Progressive degeneration of the central nervous system

between 1905 and 1965 there have been well authenticated accounts of 176 cases of 'spontaneous' regression. It is believed that these regressions were due to the immunological reaction called into action by the tumour-specific antigens. The failure to control tumour development and its growth by the body's defences can be attributed to the very slight degree of antigenicity (or foreignness) of the tumour, and to the rapid growth of the malignant tissue which overpowers the body's defence mechanism, or to impairment of this mechanism itself. The problem is how to assist man's own defence system in its response against cancer. The urgency to act in this direction is acknowledged by the World Health Organisation, which set up a committee of experts on the Immunotherapy of Cancer and recommended that 'investigations should be encouraged in the general field of tumour immunology and particularly in the development of immunotherapeutical procedures'. The investigation now in progress may find the means by which the incompatibility between cancerous growth and its victim could be increased to such a degree that immunological measures can be applied successfully.

THE FUNCTION OF GENES

Speculations as to how a gene can affect a character began soon after the discovery by Morgan and his school that genes can have more than one alternative form, or allele. By studying the various types in Drosophila, it became clear to geneticists that genes must act during embryonic life, probably in the very early stages of development. The small rudiments of wings in Drosophila were attributed to the failure of the imaginal disc in the larva to develop and differentiate into normal wings. Histological studies revealed that this is the case, but they could not throw light on the process by which the 'vestigial gene' brought about the arrest of wing development. The colour variations in the eye of Drosophila offered a more suitable material for such an investigation, as information concerning the chemistry of plant pigments was already available in the 1930s. Plant pigments were at that time considered to be valuable material of the dye-stuff industry, and their chemistry was intensively pursued. In many instances, some of the steps in the chemical reactions which led up to the final product giving the characteristic colour have been determined. Thus it was found by the biochemists that the colour varieties in the plant Primula, due to the presence of certain recessive genes, were the result of changes occurring at specific steps during the synthesis of the pigments. It was postulated that the genes, in order to produce a different colour, must alter in some manner the chemical reactions responsible for the 'normal' colour. The question is: how do genes control chemical reactions?

The first attempt to answer this question was made in 1936, when G. Beadle and B. Ephrussi carried out tests on the fruit fly, transplanting the embryonic beginning, or 'anlage', of an eye from one larva to the body cavity of another to find out if the colour of the transplanted eye could be influenced by the host. The painstaking experiments were successful; they showed that two different substances (which may be designated as A and B) are necessary to produce the normal red eye-colour. The findings also indicated that the fly with 'vermilion' eye-colour fails to produce the two substances; on the other hand, the fly with 'cinnabar' eye-colour can produce substance A but not substance B. Beadle and Ephrussi concluded that substance A is an essential precursor of substance B, which in turn is an essential precursor of the final pigment which

produces the red eye-colour of wild-type fly. It seems, therefore, that the chain reaction leading to the production of the
red pigment is interrupted at two different points: the 'vermilion' gene stops the conversion of the initial precursor
substance to substance A, while the gene 'cinnabar' acts at the
next step and blocks the conversion of substance A into B. The
process is illustrated in Fig. 24.

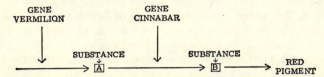

GENE
VERMILION

GENE
CINNABAR

SUBSTANCE
A

SUBSTANCE
B

RED
PIGMENT

Fig. 24. *Interference in the normal chemical reaction to
form red eye-colour resulting in vermilion or cinnabar eye-
colour in* Drosophila.

These pioneering studies showed how to tackle the problem
of gene control. However, the technical difficulties associated
with using the fruit fly prevented the extension of the work.
Real progress in this direction came when the fruit fly was
replaced by the bread mould Neurospora. Beadle, in col-
laboration with E. L. Tatum, a chemist at Stanford University,
California, determined the food requirements of this mould
and collected together a large number of 'nutritional' varieties
which were unable to synthesise food constituents and required
the addition of specific amino acids and vitamins to the culture
medium in order to exist and proliferate. These investigators
set out to identify in the different varieties of Neurospora the
'blocks' caused by genes in the synthesis of particular amino
acids.

As an example, the chain of chemical reaction resulting in
the synthesis of arginine is illustrated in Fig. 25, showing the
various steps at which the blockage occurs in different Neurospora. The 'blocks' are caused by the genes, A, B and C. C
controls the enzyme responsible for the transformation of
citrulline to arginine; B controls that which operates between
ornithine and citrulline; A directs the enzyme which trans-
forms the precursor substance into ornithine. Neurospora

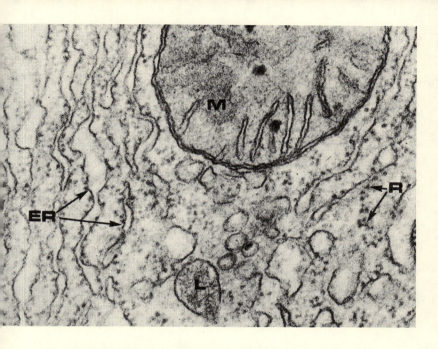

Plate I. Above: *Electron micrograph of cytoplasmic organelles in the liver cell.* M = *mitochondria;* ER = *endoplasmic reticulum;* R = *ribosomes;* L = *lysosome.* (*Magnification:* × 70 000.) Below: *Electron micrograph of the bacteriophage.* (*Magnification:* × 100 000.)

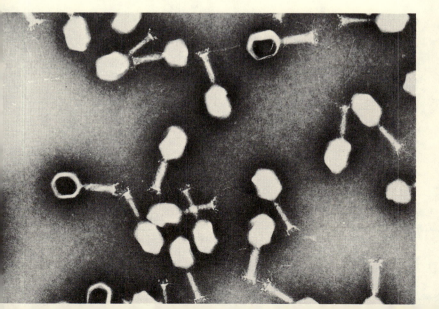

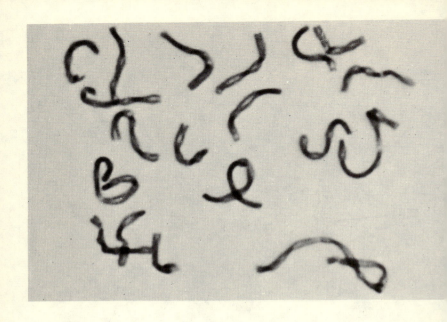

Plate II. Above:
Prophase chromosomes of a lily showing the sister chromatids.
Right: *Anaphase stage of mitosis in a cell of a fish embryo, showing the mitotic spindle.*

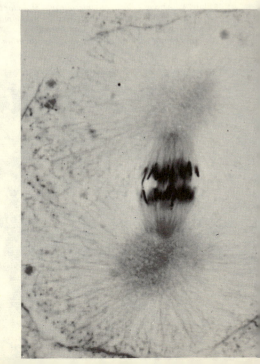

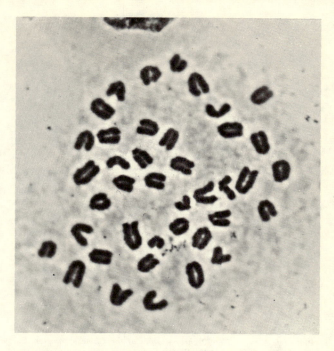

Plate III. Above: *Metaphase in a bone marrow cell of the mouse showing the 40 chromosomes.* Below: *The same in the rat, which has 42 chromosomes.*

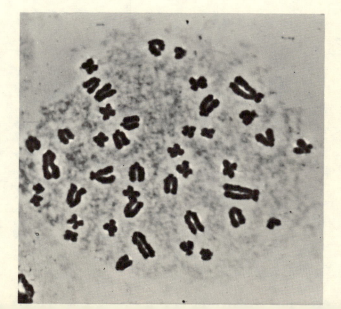

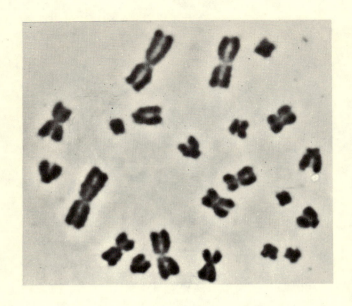

Plate IV. Above: *The 22 chromosomes of the Chinese hamster*. Below: *The 44 chromosomes of the Syrian hamster*.

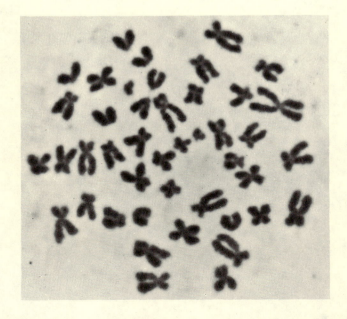

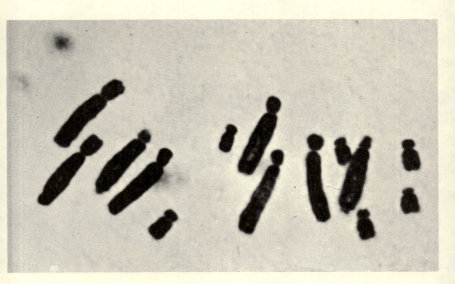

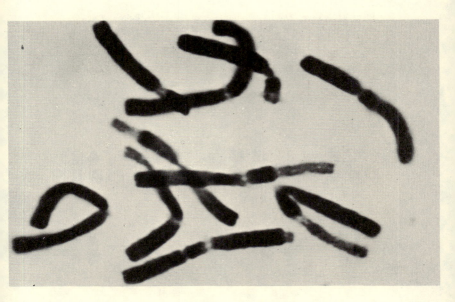

Plate V. Upper: *The 14 chromosomes of the aloe plant.* Lower: *The 10 chromosomes of a lily plant showing the heterochromatin.*

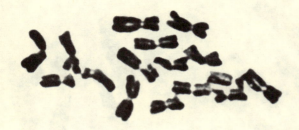

Plate VI. Above: *The 16 chromosomes of the onion.* Below: *The karyotype of the same. The chromosomes are arranged into eight pairs.*

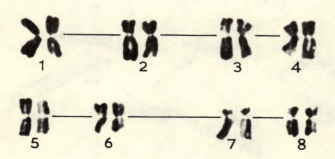

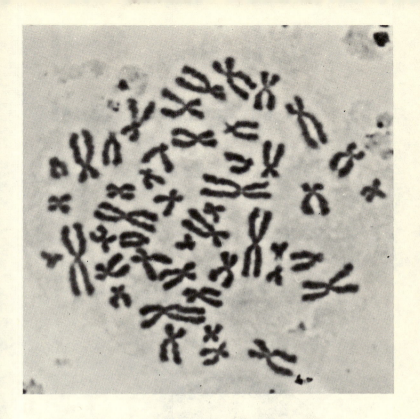

Plate VII. Above: *The 46 chromosomes of the author.* Below: *The karyotype of the same metaphase chromosomes.*

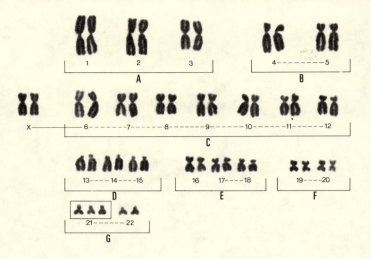

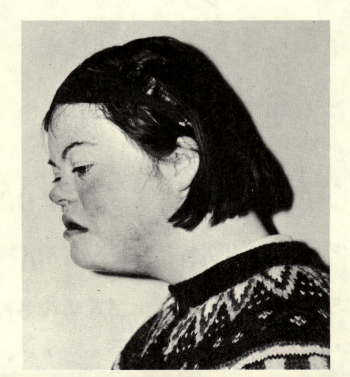

Plate VIII. Above: *The karyotype of a mongol child, showing 47 chromosomes; the extra chromosome is in the G group.* Below: *Photograph of the mongol child showing the characteristic features.*

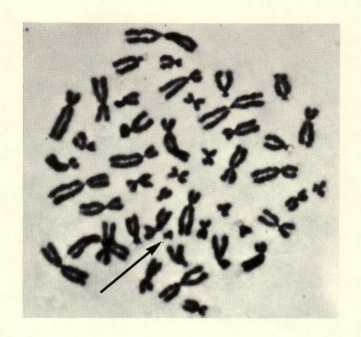

Plate IX. Above: *Metaphase in a white blood cell of a patient with chronic myeloid leukaemia, showing the abnormal chromosome no. 21 (Ph').* Below: *Karyotype of an early 'triploid' human foetus; the number of chromosomes is 69.*

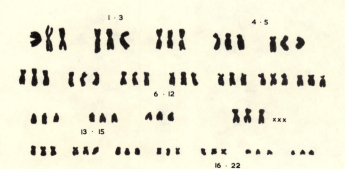

karyotype: triploid

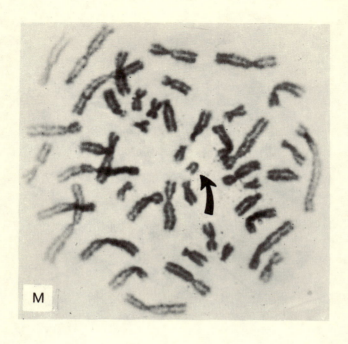

Plate X. Above: *Metaphase chromosomes in a male patient with acute lymphoid leukaemia; the abnormal chromosome no. 21 (Ch') is indicated.* Below: *The same in a female member of the same family.*

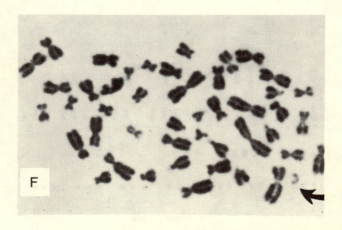

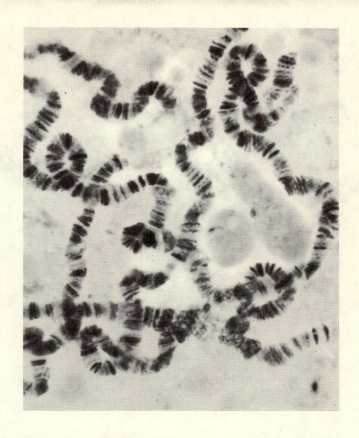

Plate XI. Above: *The giant chromosomes in the salivary gland of the fruit fly* Drosophila. Below: *Meiosis in a human male, showing the association of the sex chromosomes.*

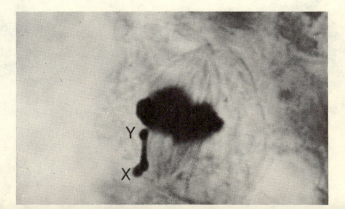

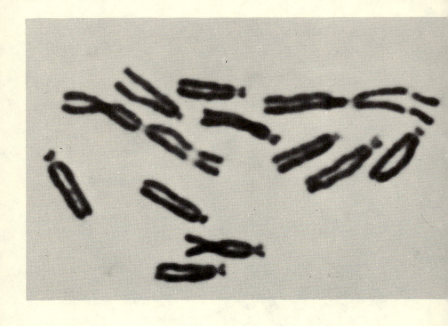

Plate XII. Above: *The 12 metaphase chromosomes of the broad bean (Vicia).* Below: *The injuries caused by irradiation to the broad bean chromosomes:* (left) *breakage followed by deletion in one chromatid;* (right) *interchange between non-homologous chromosomes.*

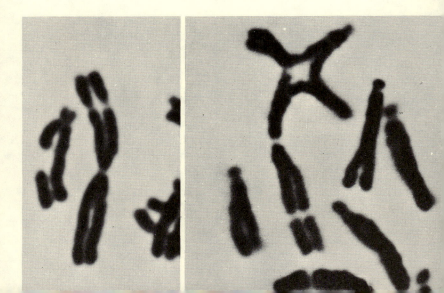

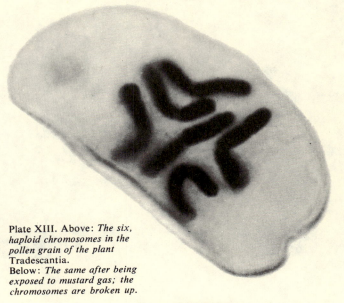

Plate XIII. Above: *The six, haploid chromosomes in the pollen grain of the plant Tradescantia.*
Below: *The same after being exposed to mustard gas; the chromosomes are broken up.*

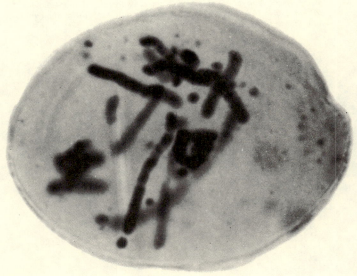

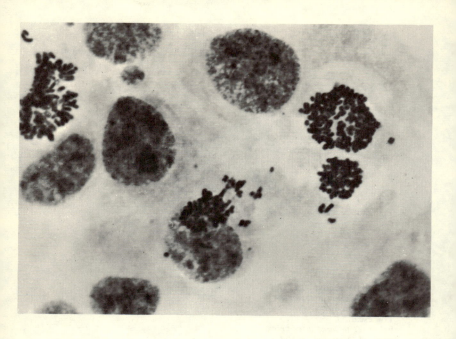

Plate XIV. Above: *Dividing cells in a cancerous tissue, showing the differences in the number of chromosomes.* Below: *Mitotic abnormalities in dividing malignant cells.*

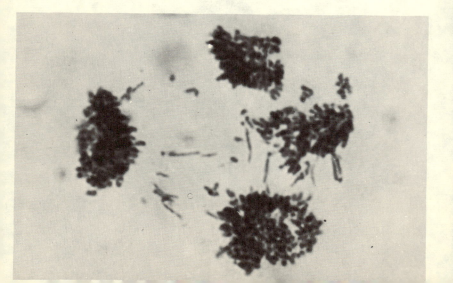

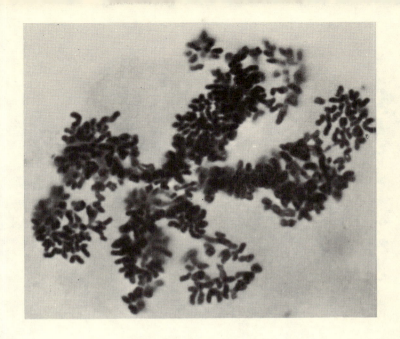

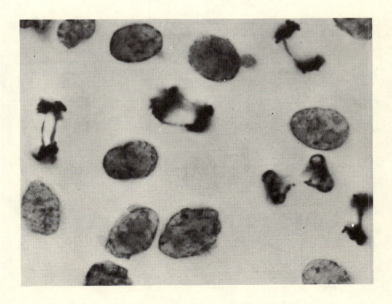

Plate XV. Upper: *Mitotic anomalies in a group of dividing malignant cells.* Lower: *Tumour in a rat, showing abnormally dividing cells.*

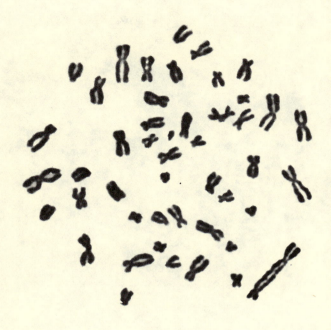

Plate XVI. Above: *48 metaphase chromosomes in a malignant cell of a patient with Burkitt lymphoma.* Below: *The karyotype of the same, showing that some chromosomes have altered structure (marker chromosomes).*

lacking the third enzyme (C-gene controlled) can only grow on the culture medium when arginine is added to it; when the second enzyme is absent, the mould requires the addition of

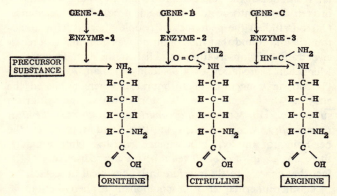

Fig. 25. *Arginine metabolism in* Neurospora; *the various 'gene-blocks' are indicated.*

citrulline and arginine; when the A-gene controlled enzyme is lacking, Neurospora would only grow when all three amino acids are added.

Many similar observations were made on nutritionally defective Neurospora, which led to the formation of the 'one gene – one enzyme' hypothesis, according to which the dominant normal gene is responsible for the enzyme present, the recessive allele for the absence of the same enzyme. When extracts were prepared from Neurospora requiring certain amino acids, it was found that the extracts lacked enzymes specific to a particular chemical reaction. This finding confirmed the 'one gene – one enzyme' hypothesis.*

Disruption of amino acid metabolism which is attributed to genes had been discovered 38 years before Beadle and Tatum made their observation in Neurospora. Sir Archibald Garrod, pathologist at St Bartholomew's Hospital, London, recorded

* What enzymes are and what they do have been discussed in a recent publication by D. W. Moss: *Enzymes* (C.S.P.15). Oliver & Boyd, 1968.

a disorder in man known as alkaptonuria, a rather rare condition in which the urine darkens on exposure to air. This change in colour was found to be due to the presence of a large amount of the acid alkapton pigment which is normally broken down into aceto-acetic acid, a colourless substance. Garrod studied the pedigrees of people affected with alkaptonuria and found that the condition was inherited as a recessive trait; this observation established the first instance of Mendelian segregation of a disability in man. According to Garrod, in congenital alkaptonuria the person lacked the enzyme which breaks the alkapton down to the colourless substance. His work, *Alkaptonuria: a study of chemical individuality*, was published in 1902 and represents the beginning of modern biochemical genetics. Unfortunately, there was a gap of over 40 years before the rediscovery of the fact that genes directly interfere in biochemical processes.

Another inherited 'error in metabolism' is phenylketonuria, a condition in which the conversion of the amino acid phenylalanine into tyrosine is blocked. The disease is more serious than alkaptonuria, as it leads to progressive mental deterioration in the affected individual. Other blocks in the metabolism of phenylalanine lead to various conditions: one is tyrosinosis, in which tyrosine metabolites are excreted in the urine; another is albinism, due to the lack of an enzyme which converts tyrosine into the pigment melanin. Albinos have colourless hair, rosy skin, pink irises, red pupils and seriously impaired vision. Fig. 26 illustrates the various blocks which can occur in the metabolism of phenylalanine.

How genes interfere in chemical reactions is beautifully illustrated in the synthesis of the amino acid histidine in the bacterium Salmonella. Biochemical studies indicated that ten enzymes are required for its synthesis. By growing Salmonella on food lacking various intermediates, ten variant types were isolated, each lacking one particular enzyme necessary for the completion of the chain reaction resulting in the formation of histidine. Genetical analysis also revealed that genes controlling the various enzymes are clustered together. By using an ingenious method, the order of the genes (numbered from 1 to

10) has been determined, each gene being responsible for the synthesis of one of the ten enzymes needed. Thus enzyme 1 is responsible for catalysing the first reaction in the synthesis, enzyme 2 for the second step, and so on.

Using Salmonella, many similar instances have been found in which genes controlling the synthesis of other amino acids also clustered together. This means that they occupy various regions along the chromosome and can be referred to as the 'histidine region', 'tryptophane region', etc. Each region contains several genes, each gene controlling a definite step in

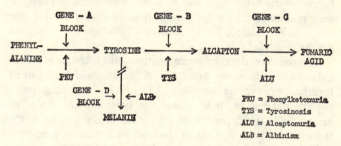

Fig. 26. *The metabolism of phenylalanine; the four 'gene-blocks' and the diseases they cause are indicated.*

the manufacture of different enzymes. The region can be looked upon as a 'super-gene' containing individual 'sub-units', or 'sites', at which specific biochemical reactions are controlled. It must be remembered that each of the 'sub-units' contributes towards the final product: one specific amino acid, e.g. arginine, or one specific protein, e.g. haemoglobin. The structural organisation and function of the 'super-gene' can be compared with the assembly line of modern factories. New discoveries in the field of biochemical genetics gave us a new concept of the gene; we now look upon it as a discrete chromosomal region consisting of units or sites arranged in linear order, each unit controlling a particular step in the synthesis of the end product. The final products are amino acids and proteins.

In nature, 20 *amino acids* are known to exist (Table 8). Some

Table 8. *Amino acids.*

Alanine (ala)	Glycine (gly)	Proline (pro)
Arginine (arg)	Histidine (his)	Serine (ser)
Asparagine (asn)	Isoleucine (ile)	Threonine (thr)
Aspartic acid (asp)	Leucine (leu)	Tryptophan (try)
Cysteine (cys)	Lysine (lys)	Tyrosine (tyr)
Glutamine (gln)	Methionine (met)	Valine (val)
Glutamic acid (glu)	Phenylalanine (phe)	

have relatively simple, others more complex structures, a factor which determines the number of enzymes required in their manufacture; e.g. for the synthesis of simple glycine one reaction is required, for the complex histidine ten reactions are necessary.

The *proteins* are even more complex, they are giant molecules in which many hundreds of amino acids are linked together by peptide bonds ($-CO-NH-$) forming polypeptide chains. In these chains the type and the order of amino acids (both controlled by genes) determine the specificity of the protein. One of the best examples of gene-controlled protein synthesis is haemoglobin, which has the capacity to bind free oxygen. For the synthesis of normal haemoglobin molecules, two distinct genes are responsible. The molecule is composed of two pairs of polypeptide chains, designated after their shape as α and β chains. A schematic representation of the haemoglobin molecule is illustrated in Fig. 27.*

It is now known that the α chain of the molecule has 141 and the β chain has 146 amino acids. In sickle-cell anaemia, in which the capacity of the red blood cell to carry oxygen is grossly impaired, the β chain differs from that in the normal haemoglobin by one of the 146 amino acids. The sequence in the corresponding sections of the two haemoglobins is as follows:

Normal (Hb-A) = val–his–leu–thr–pro–*glu*–glu–lys–
Sickle (Hb-S) = val–his–leu–thr–pro–*val*–glu–lys–

* For more detailed information about the structure of proteins, the reader is referred to *Natural High Polymers* by C. T. Greenwood and E. A. Milne (C.S.P.18). Oliver & Boyd, 1968.

All the clinical symptoms and the abnormal shape of red blood cells in sickle-cell anaemia are due to this relatively minor change concerning the replacement of glutamic acid by

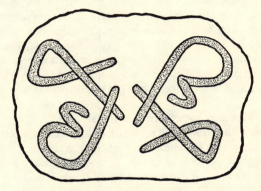

Fig. 27. *Diagram showing the two α and β chains in the haemoglobin molecule. The four chains are folded in a specific manner which is vital for the correct functioning of the molecule. The arrangement of the 'sub-units' is referred to as the 'quaternary structure'. (After Ingram, 1959.)*

valine. The disease is inherited as a Mendelian recessive, thus the change in the haemoglobin molecule reflects a permanent alteration in the gene concerned with the production of the β chain. Such a permanent change in the gene is called *mutation*. To date, more than 30 abnormal haemoglobins are known to exist in man, resulting from mutations in genes leading to changes in the amino acid sequences.

The question is: how does the mutated gene responsible for sickle-cell anaemia transfer information during haemoglobin synthesis which results in the replacement of glutamic acid with valine along the β chain? An attempt to answer this question will be made in the following section.

THE GENETIC INFORMATION IN ACTION

Sickle-cell anaemia is due to an abnormal haemoglobin, Hb-S, which differs from the normal haemoglobin by the replacement of one single amino acid in the β chain, and therefore it is often referred to as a 'molecular disease'. The Hb-S is a beautiful example in that it shows the way in which the nature of a protein molecule can be altered, and hence its specificity changed. The specificity of a protein is determined by the sequence of the amino acid components and is alone sufficient to define the structure and activity of the molecule. The primary function of genes is the 'specification' of the protein, e.g. sickle-cell gene specifies the Hb-S haemoglobin by substituting glutamic acid with valine in one of the polypeptide chain pair.

The 'sequence hypothesis', formulated in 1958 by Crick, states that 'the amino acid sequence of a protein is determined by the nucleotide sequence in a particular gene which controls that protein'. According to this theory, the genetic information is coded in the linear sequence of the purine–pyrimidine bases in the DNA molecule. As the order of bases in the polynucleotide chain determines the linear sequence of the amino acid units in the polypeptide chain of a protein, it is postulated that the component units in the two molecules must be *co-linear*, i.e. correspond to each other.

C. Yanofsky and his co-workers at Stanford University in California were the first to demonstrate such a correspondence between the genetic and protein structure. The protein studied was an enzyme present in the colon bacteria which converts indole into tryptophan, and is composed of 280 amino acids. The Stanford scientists isolated and purified six variants of this protein, each differing from the normal protein by the substitution of one single amino acid. The position of the six mutant, or sub-units, within the gene controlling the manufacture of tryptophan synthetase, and the number of amino acids separating the substitutions, showed a precise correlation.

Another evidence of co-linearity was obtained by studying a series of mutants ('amber' mutants) in T4 phage, each producing non-functional fragments of the normal protein. The investigation has been carried out in Cambridge by Crick and his associates, who similarly found a complete correspondence in the order of mutational sites of the gene and of the point of premature termination in the polypeptide chain.

These observations indicate that the genetic information coded in a segment of the DNA molecule has been transcribed, resulting in the manufacture of a particular protein in which the sequence of amino acids is related to the sequence of nucleotide bases in the DNA. The bridge between DNA and protein is the RNA, and is referred to as the 'messenger' RNA carrying the transcribed genetic code to the site where protein synthesis is taking place. The transcription occurs when the twin nucleotide strands in the DNA molecule separate and one acts as a template on which a complementary RNA strand is built. The single stranded RNA (in which the base thymine is substituted with uracil) carries the 'genetic message' to the ribosomes (subcellular organelles in the cytoplasm) on which amino acids are collected, having been formerly synthesised in the cytoplasm and transported to these sites by relatively simple RNA chains (transfer RNA). Transfer RNA (tRNA) is a relatively short molecule composed of about 77 nucleotides; there are 20 species of tRNA, one for each amino acid which is hooked on by the terminal triplet CCA. Recent studies have disclosed the mechanism by which the message from mRNA calling for the first amino acid is conveyed to the tRNA. According to the information of the messenger RNA, the amino acids are selected and linked together with peptide bonds forming polypeptide chains which are then released into the cytoplasm. Usually several ribosomes run along the messenger RNA, each contributing their amino acids for the construction of a specific protein molecule. The process is illustrated in Fig. 28.

The building blocks of proteins are provided by 20 amino acids. The question remains: what is the relationship between the four nucleotides of the DNA (adenine A, thymine T, guanine G, and cytosine C) and the amino acids? How many nucleotide bases would be required to position one individual amino acid into the messenger RNA? If we consider the four nucleotide bases as an alphabet of four letters A, T, G, and C, and the 20 amino acids as a language of 20 words, then three

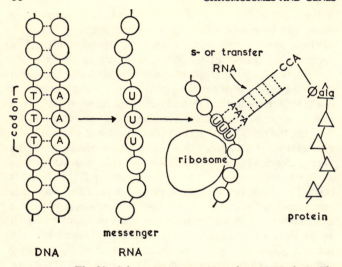

DNA   RNA

Fig. 28. *Schematic representation of protein synthesis. The triplet AAA in the DNA is transcribed as UUU to the messenger RNA; the base sequence (triplets) in the RNA is read by the ribosome which selects the appropriate transfer RNA carrying the anti-codon and corresponding amino acid (alanine) which is added to the growing polypeptide chain. Transfer RNA is a relatively short molecule composed of 77 nucleotides; there are 20 species of tRNA, one for each amino acid which is hooked on by the terminal triplet CCA. Recent studies disclosed the mechanism by which the message from mRNA calling for the first amino acid is conveyed to the appropriate tRNA.*

letters could provide 64 'code' words, more than needed to code for the 20 amino acids. These three-lettered words (triplets) are the *codons*; e.g. ATG, TGC, CAT, etc. in the DNA indicating the three adjacent nucleotide bases (i.e. ATG indicates adenine—thymine—guanine) required for selecting a particular amino acid. Table 9 shows the 64 possible combinations of the codons in the messenger RNA.

The question now is: which three-letter word, out of the possible 64, would be the code for a particular amino acid? In other words, what do the 'ATG' or 'CAT' codons in the DNA specify? It was in 1961 that the first code was identified, or 'deciphered', as the amino acid phenylalanine. The discovery was made by the biochemists M. W. Nirenberg and J. H. Matthaei at the National Institutes of Health in Washington. They used an artificial messenger RNA, composed only of uracil, synthesised originally by S. Ochoa in 1955. Nirenberg and Matthaei put the synthetic messenger RNA into 20 test-tubes, each containing all the 20 amino acids, but in each

Table 9. *The 64 possible three-letter codons in the mRNA.*

AAA	AAG	AAC	AAU
AGA	AGG	AGC	AGU
ACA	ACG	ACC	ACU
AUA	AUG	AUC	AUU
GAA	GAC	GAC	GAU
GGA	GGG	GGC	GGU
GCA	GCG	GCC	GCU
GUA	GUG	GUC	GUU
CAA	CAG	CAC	CAU
CGA	CGG	CGC	CGU
CCA	CCG	CCC	CCU
CUA	CUG	CUC	CCU
UAA	UAG	UAC	UAU
UGA	UGG	UGC	UGU
UCA	UCG	UCC	UCU
UUA	UUG	UUC	UUU

A = adenine   G = guanine   C = cytosine   U = uracil

vessel they labelled with radioactive carbon a different amino acid. The only radioactive protein formed contained the amino acid phenylalanine, indicating that the code for the protein is UUU and that the polypeptide chain is composed entirely of phenylalanine.

During the last few years, using similar methods, molecular biologists have identified the code for other amino acids, and determined the exact sequence of bases in the majority of triplets, i.e. how the letters are arranged within the 'word'. During these studies it was also discovered that more than one triplet may code for the same amino acid, e.g. the four triplets

GUU, GUC, GUA, GUG code for the amino acid valine. Table 10 lists some of the 'triplets' and the amino acids for which they code.

Table 10. *The 'triplet' code for messenger RNA.*

UUU UUC } phenylalanine	UAU UAC } tyrosine
AAA AAG } lysine	AUU AUC } isoleucine
UCU UCC AGU AGC } serine	CGC CGA AGA } arginine

The 'cracking of the genetic code' is one of the most brilliant achievements of our time. The co-operation of many scientists is yielding a rich harvest, for now we have much information concerning the nature and properties of the code. The most important characteristics of the genetic code are as follows:

(i) three adjacent nucleotide bases code for one amino acid;

(ii) any one nucleotide base takes part only in one codon;

(iii) more than one triplet can code for the same amino acid;

(iv) the code is universal, i.e. the same triplet codes for the same amino acids in different organisms.

The genes are primarily concerned in the specification of the protein structure, and the process by which the specification is achieved has been revealed. Molecular biologists are now tackling a more difficult problem: how the many kinds of protein molecules are assembled into complex structures during morphogenesis. Recent studies on the bacterial virus T4 have shown that a large number of genes are involved in the assembly of the virus particle. W. B. Wood and R. S. Edgar at the California Institute of Technology made use of mutations in those genes which control the later stages in the life cycle of T4 phage. By infecting the bacteria with different mutant viruses, they obtained incomplete virus particles: some had only a head, others only a tail or tail fibres. When these defective virus particles were mixed in a test-tube they assembled themselves in a step-by-step process to form a complete virus. Three pathways leading independently to the formation of head, tail and tail fibres were identified which combine to form the complete virus particle. These workers succeeded in localising more than 40 'morphogenetic genes' in the DNA strand of T4 phage.

When describing the Watson-Crick model of DNA, it was pointed out that the structural composition of this macro-molecule confers on it characteristics which satisfy the requirements demanded by the material basis of heredity. The two most important requirements are: (a) the structure should cater for the enormous diversity existing in the living world; and (b) the capacity to store information should be great, perhaps limitless. The present chapter described how the genetic information is stored, transcribed and translated into action, and how different proteins are produced by very simple structural changes in the DNA. This provides powerful evidence that the structural construction of DNA, as visualised by Watson and Crick in 1953, is a most suitable substance to represent the material basis of heredity.

CONTROL AND REGULATION OF GENE FUNCTION

The cells of higher organisms like man are all derived from the fertilised egg by mitosis. It is therefore assumed that the DNA, i.e. the genetic information contained in the nuclei of cells, is the same. On the other hand, while the body cells are identical in respect of their gene content (often referred to as the genome), they differ amongst themselves in shape, size and function. Our bodies are constructed from a very large number of cell types; some differentiated to do a specific job which is carried on throughout life, e.g. the nerve or muscle cells. While such cells, after being specialised for a definite function, cease to proliferate, there are others that act as 'stem cells', their function being to produce cells throughout life, e.g. cells in the basal layer of the epidermis, or in the bone marrow.

The question is when and how cells become unlike both in morphology and function. Geneticists provided proof that differentiation of cells for a particular task is directed by distinct genes during the very early stages of development. Morgan already stated in 1934 that 'different genes come into action as development proceeds'. What happens to the other genes which are also present in the nucleus? It is obvious that the activity of those genes must be restricted.

The first evidence of restricted gene function has been provided by the giant chromosomes of the secretory cells in the salivary gland of some insects (Plate XI *above*). These peculiar looking chromosomes are composed of several strands, hence they are called 'polytene' chromosomes. It has been found that certain segments of the giant chromosomes are swollen and

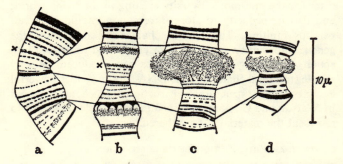

Fig. 29. *Puffing of a particular band in the polytene chromosome during different stages of development and in different tissues:* a *and* b – *larval stage,* c *and* d – *pupal stage;* a *and* c *in the Malphigian tube,* b *and* d *in the intestine. (After Beerman, 1964.)*

that these 'puffs' are sites of active RNA synthesis. That the site of the puff is actively engaged in RNA synthesis has been demonstrated by several investigators, who showed that the incorporation of labelled uridine into RNA coincides with the puffing pattern. It is believed that these sites serve as storage places for the messenger RNA. W. Beerman at the Max Planck Institute, West Germany, studying the puffing phenomenon, observed a close correlation between puffing and the developmental state of the cell; according to him, the puffing pattern of the chromosome varies from tissue to tissue and from time to time during larval development (Fig. 29).

Another example showing the restriction of gene function during development is the synthesis of haemoglobin in the human red blood cells. It has been already stated that two genes are responsible for the manufacture of the alpha and beta polypeptide chain pairs present in normal haemoglobin (Hb-A). It was discovered that in the red cells of the foetus the beta chains are missing, they are being substituted by another chain which is different in its amino acid components. This polypeptide chain (gamma chain) is a characteristic feature of the foetal haemoglobin (Hb-F) and disappears in the newborn child. It is now known that this chain is under the control of a gene that is different from those responsible for the alpha and beta chains. While the alpha chains function during foetal as well as adult life, the gene of the beta chain begins to operate around the time of birth, when the function of the gene of gamma chains declines.

Recent studies, using the methods of electrophoresis, revealed alterations in particular enzymes, the esterases, which are present in brain tissues of various mammals. It was found that the 'immature' type, A_1, pattern of the enzymes is replaced by the 'adult' type, A_2, during the later stages of embryonic development; the change occurs in the human foetus of eight months' gestation and coincides with the virtual cessation of nerve cell proliferation. This finding indicates that the gene controlling the production of the 'immature' enzyme is suppressed and at the same time the operation of another gene or sub-gene commences, resulting in the formation of the 'adult' type of esterase. It is suggested that the change represents a step necessary towards the specialised function of the nerve cells.

The examples described above show that genes can be put out of action for good. It seems that permanent suppression of genes is part of the process which results in cellular differentiation. Transplantation experiments provided evidence that this is the case in many instances. When nuclei of already differentiated cells of frog larvae are transplanted into fertilised eggs from which the nucleus has been removed previously, the development of the new embryo is grossly abnormal and has a very short life. It seems that the expression of genetic information in the nuclei of differentiated cells is restricted to a definite path, and that the part of the genome which is still active is not sufficient to promote normal development.

On the other hand, we know of many genes in plants and animals which function throughout life, but they function only when required. What is the mechanism which switches genes on and off? The problem of regulation of gene expression is the most studied one today by molecular biologists. The system chosen to study the problem is the protein synthesis in bacterial cells. These cells are known to be capable of producing hundreds or even thousands of different proteins, yet it has been found that only a very limited number is present in the cell at a given time. This observation suggests that the genes which control protein synthesis are themselves subject to some kind of direction by the cell.

The microbial system of protein synthesis, investigated by F. Jacob and J. Monod in Paris, provides a model of the possible mechanism which regulates the expression of genes. According to their scheme, the formation of polypeptide chains is initiated by a gene, the *operator* (*o*). It is postulated that the operator gene controls the function of at least two other adjacent genes, and that these genes produce messenger RNA which carries the code for the respective protein to be formed. The genes under the control of the operator are called *structural* genes, and these, together with the operator, represent a co-operative gene system called the *operon*, which is committed to make one kind of protein. The question is how or by what mechanism the operator is switched on and off to instruct the structural genes to make or not to make protein at a given time in a particular cell. According to Jacob and Monod, there are genes which regulate this process by producing a substance which represses the operator gene to initiate protein synthesis. In the colon bacteria, regulator genes have been identified and their position located in the chromosome; they act as 'repressors' or 'inducers' for enzymes involved in the synthesis of arginine, galactose, alkaline phosphatase and tryptophan, etc. It is now believed that the molecules of the repressor substance combine either with the DNA of the operator gene, thus preventing the transcription of the code on to the messenger RNA, or by blocking the attachment of the messenger RNA with the ribosomes. When the regulator gene stops producing the repressor substance, the operator gene is set free to instruct the structural genes which then could start synthesising the particular protein. Instances are known in the colon bacterium in which mutation occurred in the regulator gene, as a result of which it fails to produce the substance required to repress the operon, and the making of the respective protein is carried on whether or not it is required by the cell.

The best-studied example of gene regulation is lactose metabolism in the colon bacterium. As the pioneering work of Jacob and Monod is concerned with lactose, the system will be described in some detail. The initial steps in the metabolism of lactose involve two protein components: (i) permease, a membrane-bound protein responsible for the transport of lactose into the bacterial cell and for its concentration inside the cell; and (ii) the β-galactosidase enzyme which converts lactose into glucose and galactose. The structure of these proteins is determined by two genes, z for β-galactosidase and y for the permease. A third gene, a, was also identified which belongs to the lactose system, producing the enzyme transacetylase. The three genes lie next to one another on the chromosome, mapping in the order $z-y-a$.

The genetical information provided by the three structural genes is transcribed into the single messenger RNA (mRNA), and the information from each gene-copy within the mRNA is translated by the protein-synthesising machinery of the ribosome system into the three protein products – as indicated in Fig. 30. The synthesis of the mRNA molecule is initiated by the '*promoter*' (p), which is adjacent to or part of the gene z. The role of the promoter is to fix the rate at which the message is transcribed from genes $z-y-a$. The regulation of the lactose-structural genes is under the control of gene i, which is closely linked with the *lac*-system. The protein product of i is a

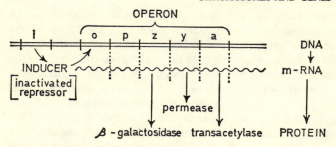

Fig. 30. *The genetic control of the synthesis of lactose in* E. coli. *(See text.)*

repressor molecule acting on the DNA of the operator (*o*) gene, inhibiting the initiation process of transcription of the code to the messenger RNA. The operator serves as a controlling site which is superimposed on the functioning unit of *z–y–a* structural genes. Intensive biochemical studies are in progress to throw more light on the nature of the binding of the repressor substance with the DNA of the operator gene on which depends a better understanding of the mechanism responsible for gene regulation.

There are several other regulatory systems which have been investigated, and in some the control is more complex than in the *lac*-system just described. J. R. Beckwith, of Harvard University at Boston, in a recent review discussed the various difficulties which have been put forward to modify the operon model, but he came to the conclusion that the evidence against the model is not strong enough to warrant modifications. The utility of Jacob-Monod's theory as a working hypothesis is unquestionable. Most studies of cell differentiation concentrate on the Jacob-Monod model, which postulates interlocked feedback processes between repressor molecules and DNA. It is expected that certain aspects of the operon model can throw some light on the more complex problems of gene regulation in cells of higher organisms. The question is: can we adapt the Jacob-Monod model to explain the complicated specialisation which characterises cell metabolism in man?

As an example illustration, we describe the synthesis of

haemoglobin, which has been analysed on the operon model by C. Baglioni. He suggests that in young human embryos the three genes responsible for the three kinds of polypeptide chains in the molecule are repressed. As development proceeds, two genes, alpha and gamma, are switched on and produce foetal haemoglobin. At a much later stage of development a third gene, beta, is switched on as well, which is followed by the repression of gene gamma and consequently by the disappearance of red cells with foetal haemoglobin. It seems that the sequence of reactions is controlled by an operon or gene-complex in which the individual components are regulated in a coordinated manner.

In haemolytic anaemia a rapid depletion of red blood cells occurs, and the need for their immediate replacement triggers off the stimulus which de-represses gene gamma and results in the synthesis of foetal haemoglobin in adult patients affected with the disease. The nature of the 'stimulus' is not known. There is some evidence that in certain instances hormones may act as inducers of protein synthesis. It is also suggested that histones, i.e. proteins bound with the DNA of chromosomes, can repress gene function and play the role of regulators.

It must be admitted that the operon model is a very simpli-fied version of the process which actually takes place in the protein-synthesising system of a mammalian cell. The exact number of proteins required for the normal functioning of a living cell is not known, but it must run to several hundreds. It is estimated that in the bacterium *E. coli*, the DNA contains the code for the sequence of amino acids in about 3000 different proteins! The proteins are formed in the cytoplasm and participate in metabolism. The chemical changes occurring in the cell altogether constitute a closely integrated system which progresses along a genetically determined path towards a specialised function. In such a system, the products of genes react with each other and the interaction plays an essential role in finalising the genetic destiny of most cells. In differentiating cells, the metabolites may act as suppressor substances for the operators of other structural genes. Automatic control of genes thus can be assured by the metabolites themselves. While the system is flexible and reversible in the bacterial cell, in the more complex system of the mammalian cell the control of repressors can be irreversible, i.e. inactivation of genes will be permanent. This might be the explanation of the fact that the transplanted 'totipotent' nucleus of the fertilised egg of the newt fails to express its 'totipotency' in the enucleated cell of the late gastrula stage; the larva is grossly abnormal and short-lived. It is likely that in the cells of the gastrula the intracellular metabolism is already fixed and the repressor substances present in the cytoplasm limit the use of the full genetic information. We can now visualise why the gene responsible for the gamma chain of foetal haemoglobin is switched off. In the newborn child a new kind of cellular metabolism takes over, and the product of this metabolism automatically represses gene gamma.

STRUCTURAL ALTERATION IN THE GENE: MUTATION

The operon model of gene regulation is accepted by many microbiologists to be one method which controls protein synthesis in bacteria and bacterial viruses. The process does not involve a change in the DNA structure, it affects only the function of the gene. When the change affects the structure of DNA, the alteration is permanent and it is multiplied by replication. Such a change is called *mutation*, it produces a new form, or allele, of a gene which by the virtue of the change acquires a new function.

In Drosophila, the normal colour of the eye in the wild-type is red; a mutation in this gene produced the white eye-colour, the first mutation to be detected by Morgan in 1909. Now we know more than 500 mutated genes in Drosophila, affecting practically every feature of the fly: the colour, shape and size of the eye; the length and number of bristles; the shape of wings; the structure of the body, etc. Similarly, there are many varieties in the bread mould Neurospora which need the addition of amino acids and vitamins to the culture medium in order to grow. In these plants the genes controlling the various enzymes which are required to complete protein synthesis have been altered and the 'faulty' genes failed to provide them. A mutation in the gene producing normal haemoglobin is the cause of the sickle-cell trait in man.

Mutations are responsible for the great variety of different individuals found within any one species, including man. In sexually reproducing organisms, following the laws of Mendel the mutant characters recombine and as a result some individuals of the species will be better adapted to a particular environment than others. The survival of the species in changing conditions may depend on such individuals. The coat colours of the hare, polar bear and tiger are the result of mutation in the gene controlling fur colour; these mutations confer the great advantage of camouflage on the animals in their struggle for survival. How natural selection acts to preserve the fit and to eliminate the unfit was documented with many examples by Charles Darwin in his book *The Origin of Species*.

We must now discuss the process of mutation at the level of the gene. According to the sequence hypothesis, 'the gene represents a region in the DNA molecule in which the sequence of the bases determines the specificity of the protein controlled by that gene'. In various ways mutation interferes with the base sequence of the DNA molecule, and, as a consequence, a different protein is produced by the mutated gene. The change in the DNA can be small or drastic and may lead to a complete loss of gene function. Basically, mutation is a chemical process, as the alteration in the gene structure consists of switching, inserting or deleting nucleotide bases in the DNA molecule. Some of the changes occur spontaneously during the replication process of the DNA when codons have been misread. 'Errors in copying' are, however, extremely rare events. The probability that such a mistake might occur in a gene is one in one hundred million (10^8) replications! On the other hand, this very low rate of mutation is sufficient to maintain the variability of the species.

A great number of physical and chemical agents are known which produce mutations at a higher rate than that of spontaneous or natural mutations. X-ray is the most powerful physical 'mutagen', a fact discovered in 1928 by H. J. Muller (see Appendix II). He exposed Drosophila to X-rays, and by applying a novel method of genetical analysis was able to detect mutations in the offspring of the irradiated male flies. Ultraviolet radiation was also soon found to be mutagenic in Drosophila as well as in plants.

The first 'chemical' mutagen was discovered in 1940 by Charlotte Auerbach at the Institute of Animal Genetics, Edinburgh. The discovery was the result of war-time research into the cell-killing property of the poison gas, sulphur mustard, used by the Germans in the First World War. The

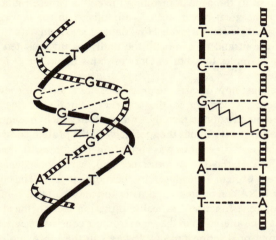

Fig. 31. *Cross-linkage between the guanine bases of the two polynucleotide chains induced by alkylating agents.*

cause of cell death was found to be damage to the chromosome mechanism of dividing cells, discovered by the author (Plate XIII). This substance, an alkylating agent, led to the synthesis of a large series of similar substances some of which are used in the therapy of cancer. Besides the alkylating agents there are many other chemical agents which are employed in mutation work (e.g. acridines, mitomycin, nitrous acid, azaserine, 2-amino purine, 5-fluorouracil, etc.). The mechanism of action of some has been revealed by biochemical studies, e.g. the alkylating agents affect DNA by cross-linking the two polynucleotide strands at the guanine base (Fig. 31); nitrous acid converts one base into another; the base analogues like 5-bromouracil are incorporated into the DNA molecule in place of thymine. Some micro-organisms, after having been exposed to chemical mutagens, become resistant to the same chemical agents. Recent studies suggest that in such instances the alterations produced in the DNA molecule are repaired by enzymes. Many mutant genes can be reverted by the same agents which were employed to produce them. In bacteria the frequency of 'forward' and 'reverse' mutation of genes is the same, in higher organisms reverse mutation is very rare.

As the genes are composed of a great number of nucleotides, mutation can affect various sites within the same gene. In the phage T4 the rII gene was found to have about 500 mutable sites – nearly half of the total length of the gene! Multiple allelism, discovered by the Morgan school, is due to multiple mutations occurring in the same gene but at different sites.

Most gene mutations are recessive and harmful, and may be lethal if the individual is homozygous for the mutated gene. In the heterozygotes the effect is usually compensated by the normal allele and cannot be detected. On the other hand, there is evidence that heterozygotes are often more fit than individuals homozygous for either the mutated or normal allele. The best example is sickle-cell anaemia. The frequency of the gene responsible for the defective haemoglobin (Hb-S) is much higher in certain parts of Africa and Southern Europe than could be expected in view of the fact that the fitness of homozygotes is zero, because they are inflicted with severe anaemia, and their reproduction rate is very low. It has been found that the heterozygotes of sickle-cell anaemia have an advantage over the homozygotes due to their resistance to malaria, caused by the Plasmodium, a parasite in the red blood cell. The resistance is due to the fact that the malaria parasites fail to complete their life cycle in the red cells of individuals heterozygous for the gene of sickle-cell anaemia.

The alteration in the structure of a gene may be very small, but the abnormal protein produced can start a chain reaction which will result in gross anomalies affecting many cells, tissues, organs and eventually the whole organism. This is particularly the case when the product of the normal allele of the gene is a protein that is essential during the earliest stages of development. A good example of such multiple, or 'pleiotropic', effect of a single gene mutation is provided by the mutant 'grey lethal' in the mouse, studied by H. Grüneberg at University College, London. The sequence of events occurring during foetal life, and the various anomalies which appear in the adult animal, are shown in Fig. 32.

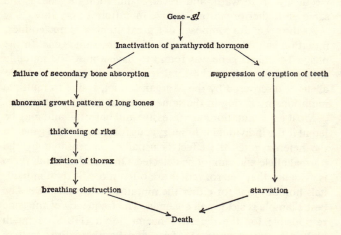

Fig. 32. *Pleiotropy or multiple effects of the gene 'grey lethal' (gl) in the mouse.*

Another example of pleiotropic effect is provided by the gene phenylketonuria, already mentioned. The condition is due to the absence of a particular enzyme as a result of which excessive amounts of phenylpyruvic acid accumulate; this affects many functions in the body, including the nervous system, and causes mental derangement.

The mutations which have been discussed represent changes within the gene and for that reason are often referred to as 'intragenic' changes. Instances are known in which a distinct region of the DNA molecule, representing one or more genes, is removed from its location to another place in the same or in a different DNA strand. When such an event occurs as the sequence of nucleotide bases remains unchanged, the function of the gene would be expected to be normal; yet observations show that the expression of the gene in the new position has been altered. The 'position effect' may be due to the influence of the new neighbour genes. The effect of the altered position on gene expression is most clearly seen when a gene is transferred to a particular chromosome region designated as the *hetero-chromatin* (Plate V). Such regions were identified in the chromosomes of Drosophila and maize, and their location has been determined. The different behaviour which these regions exhibit during the mitotic cycle indicates an unusual type of organisation and function.

A very interesting phenomenon, in which pieces of chromosomes are transferred not within but between different cells, has been discovered in the bacterium Salmonella. The transfer takes place by the help of a special type of bacteria virus, the temperate phage. This virus infects Salmonella and multiplies inside without interfering with the host, which is able to divide in spite of the presence of the phage. During the division of the Salmonella the phage picks up a segment of the replicating bacterial DNA. When Salmonella is destroyed by lysis (dissolution of the bacterial envelope) the phage carrying bacterial DNA is liberated and is ready to infect other Salmonellae. When this takes place, the piece of DNA molecule of the previous host is detached from the phage and incorporated into the DNA of the new host. The phenomenon is called *transduction*; by this process gene or genes of one bacterium can be 'transducted' into another. It has been demonstrated that in this way the mutant gene responsible for streptomycin resistance could be transferred. The incorporation of a 'transducted' segment of DNA into the DNA of the recipient is another way to confer new genetic characters on bacteria.

Mutation is not restricted to particular cells or tissues; it can also occur at any time during the life of the organism. Mutation in genes carried by the gametes (germinal mutation) can be transmitted to a new individual at fertilisation. In this case, every cell of the embryo will contain the mutated gene. On the other hand, when mutation occurs after fertilisation (somatic mutation), the mutated gene is restricted to the descendants of the cell in which it took place. If somatic mutation occurs during the very early stages of embryonic development, it may be detected by a different appearance of certain regions in the body of the adult. The variegated patterns of leaves or flowers of plants are due to such mutations. A light streak in dark hair, and a brown segment in an otherwise blue iris in the eye, are examples of somatic mutation in man. The phenomenon is known as 'mosaicism' and is characterised by the presence of genetically different tissues in the *same* organism. Mosaicism can be the result of gene mutation; it can also be brought about by loss or addition of chromosome regions or of whole chromosomes. The discussion of the genetical effects due to gross chromosomal changes is the subject of the next chapter.

4. Cytogenetics: The Study of Chromosome Behaviour

Chromosomes are the material basis of heredity and variation, through them is transmitted the blue-print of the genetic information from cell to cell, from parents to offspring. It was around 1920 that Morgan and his followers put forward in a definite form the chromosome theory of heredity. Their ideas were supported by E. B. Wilson at Columbia University, New York, who collected together many observations from cytological studies, indicating the important role of chromosomes in hereditary transmission. In his *Recent Advances in Cytology*, C. D. Darlington of the John Innes Horticultural Institute, London, brought together an impressive amount of information concerning chromosome behaviour in both plants and animals. Much of this information has been obtained by his own brilliant studies. Darlington demonstrated convincingly that by studying chromosome behaviour alone, the genetic behaviour of the organism can be inferred and predicted. He is considered to be the founder of the new discipline: *cytogenetics*, the study of chromosome behaviour.

The following section describes some of the important findings of cytogenetic studies with special reference to man.

CHROMOSOMAL CHANGES AND THEIR CONSEQUENCE

It has been argued that normal development and functioning of an organism depends on the interaction of genes. As genes are located at well-defined positions in the chromosomes, anomalies which involve the chromosomes can be expected to cause disturbances in the expression of the genes. The consequence is very often an unusual type of heredity, the

appearance of morphological abnormality or malfunctioning
of physiological systems in the affected organism.

Cytological studies revealed two kinds of chromosome
anomalies; one concerns the number, the other the structure of
chromosomes.

The most simple *numerical* alteration is when only one
chromosome is involved; it is either added to or lost from the
normal chromosome set. The process responsible is known as
chromosome 'non-disjunction', which takes place during
gamete formation. The first such case has been observed in
Drosophila, and because of its importance, is discussed here
in more detail.

The unusual inheritance of the sex-linked gene (*y*) responsible for the yellow body-colour encountered by Morgan in
one of his experiments indicated that it might be caused by a
chromosome anomaly. According to the rule of sex-linked
inheritance, the recessive gene of yellow is transmitted from
mothers to their sons. In the case mentioned, the daughters
instead of the sons had the yellow body, the sons were all
wild-type like their father! Examination of the chromosomes
revealed that the daughters had two X chromosomes attached
to each other, each X carrying the gene *y* for yellow body-colour, and in addition they also had a Y chromosome; thus in
these flies the number of chromosomes was nine instead of the
normal eight. The chromosome constitutions of the mother,
father and that of the gametes, and the genetic consequences of
the anomaly, are illustrated in Fig. 33. The diagram shows
that the segregation of the anomalous chromosomes results not
only in an unexpected transmission of the yellow body-colour,
but that it also causes the death of 50 per cent of the male
offspring; those eggs which have a Y chromosome fail to hatch
when fertilised by a sperm carrying a Y chromosome. The
diagram also shows that in respect of chromosome constitution, the daughters are of two kinds: half of the daughters are
like their mother ($\overline{XX}$ Y), the other half have three Xes
($\overline{XX}$ X) – two being attached, derived from the mother, the
third contributed by the father. Such females do not breed,
they are sterile.

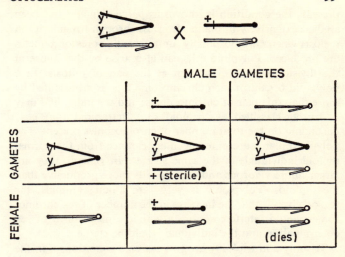

Fig. 33. *Non-disjunction of the two attached X chromosomes in* Drosophila, *and its consequence in heredity.*

The first instance of a numerical change in chromosome constitution revealed three phenomena: (i) irregularity in hereditary transmission, (ii) intereference with viability, and (iii) interference with the physiology of the affected organism.

The Drosophila case of non-disjunction is unusual in that the chromosome anomaly was brought about by the attachment of the two sex chromosomes. In most instances in which anomalies in the number of chromosomes were observed, they were not attached but were free from each other. The condition in which one extra chromosome is present is called *trisomy*: in such conditions a particular chromosome has *three* representatives instead of the usual two. The best example of trisomy is provided by the plant Jimson weed. As the normal plant has 12 pairs of chromosomes, 12 different trisomic types are possible, each with an extra member of a different chromosome pair which produces distinctive characteristics, affecting the shape of fruit, leaves and vigour of the plant.

Often more than two complete sets of chromosomes are

present; the condition is known as *polyploidy* and has been studied extensively in plants. It arises through irregularity in meiosis when chromosomally 'un-reduced' spores or gametes are produced. Polyploid cells can also arise by the failure of the division of cell cytoplasm at the end of mitosis. In a polyploid organism each chromosome type is represented by more than one pair of chromosomes; and the individual may be further classified as 'triploid' (3*n*), 'tetraploid' (4*n*), etc., depending on the total number of chromosomes present. The polyploid plants are different in appearance from the normal diploid individuals of the same species. In general, they are larger, more vigorous and occasionally more productive than the diploids. Polyploidy is very rare among animals, the reason given is that the increase in the number of sex chromosomes would interfere seriously with the mechanism of sex determination and the individual would be sterile.

Trisomy and triploidy are two extreme conditions – in the former only one extra chromosome is present, in the latter every chromosome type has an extra member. Between these conditions there are alterations in chromosome number when more than one chromosome type is affected; such a situation is designated as *aneuploidy*.

Changes affecting the *structure* of chromosomes are: (i) deletion, (ii) duplication, (iii) inversion and (iv) translocation.

(i) Deletion consists of loss of part of a chromosome; if the region is large, it may cause the death of the individual. Small deletions survive and prove very useful in mapping the position of genes in the chromosomes. Loss of a definite segment of a chromosome removes the genes within the segment, and permits, in a heterozygous individual, the manifestation of characters which are determined by recessive genes. By using deletions the position of many genes were accurately determined in the giant chromosomes of the salivary gland of Drosophila. Similarly, to locate genes in the chromosomes of the colon bacterium, deletions were used extensively. Although individuals with losses of short chromosome segments are viable, there is usually a marked effect on particular developmental reactions. Homozygous deletions are lethal, which is a further proof that the entire genetic material is essential for life and normal development. When both ends of a chromosome have been lost, the broken end may rejoin and a ring-shaped chromosome is formed. The 'ring-chromosome' can replicate, but very often it undergoes further structural alteration and is eliminated.

(ii) Duplication consists of the presence of an additional piece of chromosome material. This condition may be considered to be a special type of trisomy in which a very small chromosome region is involved. Duplications were found to be less harmful to the organism than deletions. The effects they produce are related to length; long pieces have greater effect than short ones. Duplicated segments carrying the wild-type genes make the recessive alleles present in the corresponding chromosome region ineffective. In such a situation, duplications act as suppressors of recessive traits. Duplications were identified in Drosophila and micro-organisms which are located next to the original position of the particular chromosome region. Such duplications are referred to as 'repeats'. It is more than likely that a shift in the position of the paired chromosomes during meiosis results in 'unequal crossing-over' and that this event is responsible for the 'repeats'. The mutant Bar and double-Bar genes, affecting the size and shape of the eye in Drosophila, are good examples. The 'repeats' are believed to be a mechanism by which new genes are acquired during the evolution of species.

(iii) Inversion represents an alteration which affects the sequence of genes in the chromosome. In an individual heterozygous for an inversion, the alteration interferes with the pairing of homologous chromosomes during meiosis. It has been found that crossing-over between the 'inverted' and normal chromosomes produces chromosomally abnormal, non-viable gametes. Another consequence of inversion is a reduction in the frequency of crossing-over within the inverted chromosome region. Genes located in this segment are inherited together and in certain situations this may represent an advantage for the species.

(iv) Translocation consists of transferring a chromosome region into another chromosome. Such changes are usually reciprocal, i.e. the segments are exchanged between two chromosomes. As a result, genes in the translocated segments will be linked to the genes present in the recipient chromosome. The individual carrying a reciprocal translocation is usually normal, as the entire chromosome material is present, although it may be differently arranged. The effect of chromosome translocation becomes manifest only during meiosis. The association and segregation of the four chromosomes, two of which contain the translocated segments, produce in respect of the chromosome content, balanced and unbalanced gametes. Chromosome unbalance is due to excessive deficiency or duplication of chromosome material. When such an unbalanced gamete fertilises a normal gamete, the fertilised egg is non-viable. Reduced fertility, often referred to as 'semi-sterility', indicates that the organism is a translocation carrier.

Another type of structural change is brought about by 'mis-division' of the centrome, which at the end of metaphase splits transversely instead of longitudinally to the axis of the chromosome. The result is two 'iso-chromosomes'; each is composed of two identical halfs, one chromosome arm is present in duplicate and the other arm is missing. These chromosomes, in comparison with normal ones, are partly duplications and partly deficiencies.

Extensive cytological and genetical studies of the numerical and structural changes of chromosomes have been carried out in plants and animals, and the knowledge gained from these studies has helped us in recent years to identify and interpret the cause of many congenital anomalies in man himself.

CHROMOSOME ANOMALIES IN MAN

In view of the fact that many developmental abnormalities in plants and animals have been found to be due to chromosomal anomalies, geneticists began to consider in the early 1930s the possibility that certain aberrations of human development may be associated with chromosome abnormalities. In 1932 Haldane had suggested that aberrations in human sex differentiation might have a chromosomal basis. Similarly, and at the same time, chromosome irregularity was considered by P. J. Waardenburg in Holland and by L. S. Penrose in England to be the cause of 'mongolism', a condition characterised by facial features resembling slightly those found in the Asiatic tribe of Mongols.

The syndrome has been known since 1866, when Langdon Haydon Down described it. He was the Superintendent of the Earlswood Asylum for Idiots in Surrey and had much opportunity to observe the 'mongolian' type of mentally handicapped children. According to the first account of mongolism, 'The hair of the affected child is not black as in the real Mongol but of a brownish colour, straight and scanty. The face is flat and broad and destitute of prominence. The cheeks are roundish and extended laterally. The eyes are obliquely placed, and the internal canthi more than normally distant from one another. The forehead is wrinkled from the constant use of the muscles to assist in the opening of the eyes. The lips are large and thick, much roughened and the nose is small. The skin has a dirty yellowish tinge and is deficient in elasticity, giving the appearance of being too large for the body' (Plate VIII *above*). Down recognised that some unusual pathological process is at work in the mentally retarded and physically grossly abnormal 'mongol' children.

The cause of 'Down's syndrome', as it is now called, remained unknown for nearly 100 years. The incidence of 'mongols' in certain families, the association of the birth of children showing the syndrome with advanced age of the mother, and the 50 or more separate clinical features indicated that the condition could not be due to one gene only. In a 'mongol', practically every tissue of the body is affected; thus the cells are of abnormal dimensions and, during foetal development, are imperfectly synchronised; the basal metabolism is low; the function of pituitary and thyroid glands is abnormal; glucose tolerance is variable; the calcium content of the blood is low; the segmentation of the nucleus in the white blood cells is diminished, etc. The evidence that the cause of Down's syndrome is a chromosome anomaly was provided by three French scientists, J. M. Lejeune, M. Gautier and R. Turpin. They reported in 1959 that the number of chromosomes in persons with this syndrome is 47 instead of 46 and that the extra chromosome present in the cells is chromosome no. 21 of the G group. Their findings were verified soon after, both in Great Britain and in the United States; thus Waardenburg's suggestion put forward two decades previously, that the condition might be due to chromosome irregularity, has been confirmed. Now it is accepted that Down's syndrome is caused by the trisomy of chromosome no. 21 (Plate VIII *above*).

The incidence of children born with the Down's syndrome is estimated to be about 1 in 700 live births, but it was found that the risk of having such a child increases with the age of the mother: when the age of the mother is between 30–34 years, the risk is 1 in 600–700 births; it is 1 in 70 when the mother's age is between 40–45 years (Fig. 34).

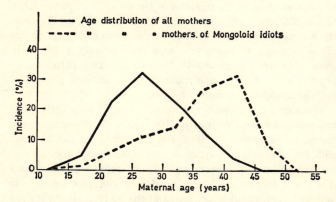

Fig. 34. *Graph showing the age of mothers of mongol children as compared with the age of mothers in the control group.*

The cytological studies of patients with Down's syndrome revealed a number of different chromosome anomalies which are associated with the same condition. All of them, can, however, be interpreted as instances of excess material belonging to chromosome no. 21. It was found that the extra chromosome material is inserted or attached to a chromosome of the D group (numbers 13–15) or to the other chromosome of the G group (chromosome no. 22), thus although the chromosome number is 46, chromosome no. 21 is present in excess.

The first case of a '46-chromosome, or translocation, mongol' was reported in 1960 by P. E. Polani and his associates. Their finding is very important for two reasons, it explains (i) why Down's syndrome is inherited in certain families and (ii) why the age of the mother is lower in these families than the average age of mothers of the 'trisomic' mongol children. According to Penrose, the average age of the latter is 38 years, that of the former is 28; these mothers are carriers of a chromosome 21 translocation. In familial Down's syndrome, differences were observed in the extent of mental retardation shown by the mongol child; it is probably related to the size of the translocated segments.

Although we know that Down's syndrome is associated with the presence of extra chromosomal material, we still do not know what causes the cytological anomaly. One of the most important findings is that the non-disjunction of chromosome 21 during meiosis occurs more frequently in older mothers than in young ones.

Penrose advanced the hypothesis that recessive genes in the mother might be responsible for causing non-disjunction of chromosome 21. Such an instance is known in the fruit fly Drosophila. Occasional appearances together of two kinds of trisomy, when two different chromosomes are present in triplicate in the same person, seemed to indicate that one of the parents had inherited the tendency to chromosomal non-disjunction. Studies of first-cousin marriages showed, however, that mongolism is not more common in these than in other marriages, and other investigations also failed to support the hypothesis that Down's syndrome is the indirect result of the operation of recessive genes which affect chromosome separation during meiosis.

Two other trisomic conditions have been described in man:

in one the extra chromosome belongs to the E group (possibly chromosome no. 18), in the other it belongs to the D group (chromosomes no. 13–15). The symptoms of E-trisomy are severe, and children born with it rarely survive beyond six months. D-trisomy is associated with multiple developmental anomalies, including cleft palate and lip, extra fingers and toes. Table 11 summarises the most important features of the three chromosome trisomies.

Table 11. *Autosomal trisomy syndromes.*

Chromosome anomaly	Pathological anomalies*
D-trisomy (13–15)	Eye defects, deafness. polydactyly, cleft palate, seizures, haemangioma, hare lip, anomalous palmar creases, interventricular septal defect, mental retardation
E-trisomy (18)	Failure to thrive, malformed ear, micrognathia, hernia, hypertonicity, defective ossification of sternum, flexion fingers, hip abduction, mental retardation
21-trisomy	Short stature, small round head, protruding fissured tongue, abnormal thyroid function, anomalous dermatoglyphic patterns, immature leukocytes in blood, prevalence to leukaemia in childhood, decreased blood-calcium levels, mental retardation

* Compiled from reports of several authors.

Congenital anomalies are also known which are due to irregularities not in the autosomal but in the sex chromosome constitution; the best-known are Turner's and Klinefelter's syndromes. The former is due to the loss of one X or Y chromosome; the patient has only 45 chromosomes and an XO sex chromosome constitution. The internal sex organs of such a person are female, which, however, failed to differentiate and function; the breasts are poorly developed, and the external genitalia remain juvenile. Individuals with Turner's syndrome are usually brought up as girls until puberty, as they show only slight anomalies before this age. The frequency of this syndrome is 1 in 3000 live births.

Klinefelter's syndrome is due to the presence of an extra X chromosome; the patient has 47 chromosomes and an XXY sex chromosome constitution. Many of the affected males are mentally retarded, have small testes and show female development of the breast.

Since the recognition of chromosomal abnormalities in Down's, Turner's and Klinefelter's syndromes, many more chromosome anomalies have been observed. Table 12 shows

Table 12. *Alterations in chromosome number.*

Number observed	Chromosome constitution	Syndrome
45	44a* + XO	Turner's syndrome (female appearance) (1/5000)†
47	44a + XXX	Ovarian hypofunction (mild mental defect?) (1/1500)
	44a + XXY	Klinefelter's syndrome (male appearance) (1/750)
	46 + C(6–12)	Mental deficiency
	46 + D(13–15)	D-trisomy syndrome Multiple anomalies
	46 + E(16–18)	E-trisomy syndrome Multiple anomalies
	46 + G (21)	Down's syndrome (mongolism)
48	44a + XXXX	Mentally defective
	44a + G(21) + XXY	Down's + Klinefelter's syndromes
49	44a + XXXXY	Mental retardation Skeletal defects Sex defects

* a = autosomes.
† Incidence of persons born with syndrome.

some examples of numerical changes in the chromosome constitution of man. Many produce both physical and mental disabilities.

Recent studies indicate that chromosome anomaly might be associated with a tendency for delinquency and crime. A

survey at a special security hospital in Scotland for danger-
ously violent and criminal patients demonstrated such a link.
A group of patients has been found to have two Y chromosomes instead of the normal one, their sex chromosome constitution is XYY. Such patients are unusually tall (6 ft or more)
but otherwise physically normal, show gross disturbance in
personality and temperament and come into conflict with the
law at a very early age. The XYY men are first convicted on
average at 13, the XY control group at 18 years of age; the
offences of the former group are against property and not
against people. Table 13 shows the difference between XYY
and XY patients.

Table 13. *The type and frequency of criminal offences in
eight XYY individuals and 18 controls.*

	XYY	XY
Offences against persons	8·7%	21·9%
Offences against property	88·3%	62·9%
Average age at first crime	13 years	18 years

A similar observation was made in a London prison: 2 out of
34 convicts whose height was 6 ft or more had XYY chromosome constitution; one had an unusually large Y chromosome.
The observations of British scientists have been confirmed by
Dr Mary Telfer and her colleagues at the Elwyn Institute,
Pennsylvania. They examined the chromosomes of 129 male
patients over 6 ft tall at four institutions for the detention of
criminals and found that 5 had 47 chromosomes with XYY sex
chromosome constitution.

According to Dr W. H. Price and Dr P. B. Whatmore, the
XYY men suffer from severe disturbance of the whole
personality, showing extreme instability and irresponsibility
with lack of affection for others, and being incapable of
tolerating frustration. The findings of these scientists raise
important questions about the extent to which people with
such abnormalities ought to be held responsible for their
deeds. If the XYY man cannot help being a criminal because

of his extra Y chromosome, what kind of corrective measure should be applied to him? How can we rehabilitate such a person into society? These are problems for which sociologists must find a solution. The first task is to find out what proportion of our prison population has chromosomal anomaly and then what is the frequency of this and similar chromosome defects in the population at large.

The numerical alterations are relatively easy to detect in human; more difficulty is encountered in recognising *structural* changes in the chromosomes. Search for such abnormalities is going on, and some of the structural changes so far identified are given in Table 14.

Table 14. *Alterations in chromosome structure.*

Type of change	Chromosomes involved	Syndrome
Translocation	no. 21– no. 15	Down's syndrome
	no. 22– no. 13	Mental deficiency
		Heart disease
	no. 2 – no. 2	Waldenström's macroglobulinaemia
	X–X(?)	Amenorrhoea*
Deletion	Long arm of X	Oligomenorrhoea†
	Short arm of X	Amenorrhoea
	no. 21 (PH′)	Chronic myeloid leukaemia
Duplication (partial trisomy)	no. 2 (iso-chromosome)	Waldenström's macroglobulinaemia
	X (long arm)	Amenorrhoea
	no. 22	Sturge-Weber's syndrome
Inversion	no. 21	Down's syndrome

* Absence of menstruation.
† Irregular menstruation.

Structural changes are specially important when the gametes carrying the altered chromosomes are viable and can be transmitted from parents to offspring. The children who receive such altered chromosomes may exhibit serious developmental abnormalities. The first structural change observed was that of the translocation of chromosome no. 21, responsible for the familial incidence of Down's syndrome. Recently it was reported that a mentally retarded boy and a mentally retarded girl in a Derby Children's Hospital both had structurally altered chromosomes. The cytological analysis revealed that their mother was a carrier of a balanced translocation which involved chromosomes belonging to C and D groups. A ring chromosome was found in another mentally retarded patient, the chromosome being identified was one of the D group.

The '*Cri du chat*' syndrome is another condition, due to structural change consisting of a deletion in a chromosome of group B. The chromosome involved is broken, and when the broken ends reunite it forms a ring structure. The syndrome got its name from the peculiar sound resembling that of a cat which the child makes at birth. Such patients show mental retardation, several minor skeletal abnormalities and heart defects. The first case was recognised in 1963 in France, since then several other cases have been reported in Britain and in the United States.

The 'pericentric syndrome' is associated with an inversion including the centromere in a chromosome belonging to the C group; the syndrome consists of mental retardation, microcephaly (small head), abnormal slit palate and vision.

The finding of chromosome abnormalities in children with congenital syndromes very often resulting in early death, suggested the possibility of finding gross chromosomal anomalies in abortuses and still-born infants. Systemic study has been undertaken by D. H. Carr in Canada. His report, published in 1963, provided valuable information on this subject, showing that chromosomal abnormalities are a significant cause of early embryonic death. The interest aroused by his report has initiated more studies, the results of which were summarised at a conference held in Geneva by the World Health Organisation in 1966. The survey covered 450 induced and 800 spontaneous abortions, and on the basis of the available data some tentative conclusions have been reached at the Conference.

The survey revealed that chromosome anomalies are more frequent in spontaneous than in induced abortions; 19 per cent were observed in the former group, and only 2 per cent in the latter. It was found that 21 per cent of the foetuses lost one chromosome from the C group, believed to be the sex chromosome. The most common type of chromosome anomaly observed in aborted foetuses was the addition of an extra chromosome to the genome. The extra, or trisomic, chromosome was identified as a chromosome belonging to the D, E or G group. Triploidy (3*n*) consisting of 69 chromosomes was present in 17 per cent of the abortuses (Plate IX *above*). The data also suggested that more females than male foetuses are aborted. The survey covered instances of habitual aborters and found that abnormalities in the parental chromosomes play a significant role in recurrent abortion and that the risk of having spontaneous abortion is increased when the mother has previously had an abortion.

The cases studied by Carr seem to indicate that maternal age has some influence on producing chromosome anomalies and causing the death of the foetus, the critical age is between 34 and 47 years. One case reported by him is of special interest. The mother was 35 years of age when her twin foetuses aborted; she had already had an abortion previously. One of the twin foetuses had an extra trisomic chromosome, the other was triploid – having 69 chromosomes in every cell analysed.

The frequency of chromosomal changes in 72 spontaneous abortions, pooled from six sources, is shown in Table 15. The

Table 15. *Chromosome studies in abortions.*

Induced	Spontaneous	Authors	
127	—	Makino (1962)	
—	200	Carr (1963, 1965)	
—	10	Clendenin (1963)	
—	8	Hall (1964)	
8	12	Thiede (1964)	
15	25	Szulman (1965)	
29	6	Klinger (1965)	
179	261	TOTAL	
175	189	Normal	} Chromosome
4	72	Abnormal	∫ constitution
(2·26%)	(27·58%)		

types of the anomalies were analysed by P. E. Polani, who found that 20 per cent of the aborted foetuses were triploid (3n), 4 per cent tetraploid (4n), and 3 per cent grossly aneuploid. The ratio of autosomal to sex chromosome anomalies in abortions is 2:1, in live births the ratio is 1:1, which suggests that anomalies involving the sex chromosomes are better tolerated than those affecting the autosomes.

The studies so far available show that nearly a fourth or perhaps even a higher proportion of early spontaneous human abortions carry chromosome anomalies, causing the death of the foetus.

At present, the main aim of cytogenetic studies of congenital malformations is to clarify the possible chromosomal basis of a particular syndrome. Towards this aim much valuable information has already been accumulated and used in clinical practice, e.g. diagnosing the genetic sex in the various intersex states and giving reliable prognosis in the case of familial Down's syndrome. Chromosome anomalies can also help in revealing the gene content of a particular chromosome or chromosome region. Such studies have been made with great success in animals (Drosophila, the mouse), plants (maize) and micro-organisms (*E. coli*), the information gained making possible the construction of genetic maps. Genetic mapping in man has, however, been delayed and will remain so until the identification of individual chromosomes becomes more accurate. By considering both genetical and cytological methods, a start has been made towards localising genes. It is known that the human X chromosome carries the genes governing a blood group, haemophilia, red–green colourblindness, glucose-6-phosphate dehydrogenase, muscular dystrophy, height and gonadal development. The gene of retinoblastoma (cancer of the eye) is located in chromosome no. 15. The exact localisation of genes responsible for the synthesis of haemoglobin in the red blood cell may be possible in the future by the use of particular chromosome anomalies already mentioned. It seems that the genes are located in a chromosome of group D.

It is more or less a common experience of the geneticists that gross chromosome anomalies such as E or D trisomies affect a great many tissues and organs in the body, and that the extent of the physical and mental anomalies varies in different individuals. Could it be assumed that those genes which control development and differentiation of these tissues and organs are located in the particular chromosome which is involved in the anomaly? Or should we rather attribute the wide spectrum of the syndrome to the gross interference with the internal balance of the whole genome? New chromosome aberrations are reported almost daily. Numerous deletions, duplications, inversions, reciprocal translocations, ring chromosomes, single and double trisomies, triploidy, and tetraploidy have so far been identified and the genetical consequences analysed. The intensive cytogenetical studies in progress all over the world should eventually provide the information needed towards the mapping of genes in the chromosomes of man.

CHROMOSOMAL MOSAICISM

The various numerical and structural anomalies discussed previously are present in every cell of the affected individual. It is believed that such chromosome anomalies are originated during gametogenesis and are transmitted through the egg or sperm to the new individual in which all the cells contain the same chromosome anomaly. Chromosomal changes, however, can be brought about by disturbances in the process of cell division after fertilisation. Many instances are now known where irregular mitosis, particularly chromosome non-disjunction, occurs during embryonic development and even in adult life. The individual in which such an event has taken place has in the cells of various tissues different chromosome numbers, i.e. an altered genome. The irregularities arising during foetal life or in the adult are considered under the heading of 'chromosomal mosaicism'.

Chromosomal mosaicism was first detected in a patient with Klinefelter's syndrome. In this person most of the blood cells had 47 chromosomes – 44 autosomes and XXY sex chromosome – which is the characteristic chromosome constitution in

Klinefelter's syndrome. Beside the chromosomally abnormal cells, there were also cells in the blood with the normal chromosome number and sex chromosome constitution (44 autosomes and XX). It was clear that this patient had two cell lines: one with the normal 46 chromosomes and another with 47, the two differing in respect of the sex chromosome constitution (XX/XXY mosaicism). Instances were also found in which more than two different cell lines were present.

Mosaicism is more frequent in persons who already have chromosome anomaly, which they inherited or acquired at fertilisation. Such a case was reported from Switzerland. A physically abnormal and mentally deficient 11-month-old boy had two cell lines: while the cells in the blood had 48 chromosomes, cells of the skin were of two kinds, one had 48 and the other 71 chromosomes. The 48-chromosome cells in the blood and skin had XXYY, those with 71 had XXXYY sex chromosome constitution. Normal cells with 46 chromosomes were absent from the tissues analysed. It is assumed that the first chromosome anomaly occurred at fertilisation and was followed by another which took place at a later stage of embryonic development.

Another kind of mosaicism has been described from British Columbia. A seven-year-old 'boy', who was born with abnormal genitalia, showed variable patches of pigmentation in his skin, an unusual combination of blood groups and serum proteins. Cytological analysis revealed that all his cells studied had the normal chromosome number, i.e. 46. Further scrutiny, however, showed that these cells were of two kinds; one had XX and the other XY sex chromosomes, i.e. one cell population was female, the other male! In the blood, the proportion of the female (XX) cells was 60 per cent, in the excised ovarian tissue 100 per cent. The proportion of male (XY) cells in the skin varied between 6 and 40 per cent. The case is of special interest, for it is an instance in which the fertilisation of the egg by two sperms (one with X, the other with Y chromosome) was followed by another mitotic anomaly occurring at the very early cleavage division. Some examples of sex chromosome mosaicism and the pathological syndromes associated with the anomalies are given in Table 16.

Mosaicism involving the autosome chromosomes can also occur, though the event is very rare. A case of autosomal

Table 16. *Sex chromosome mosaics.*

Constitution	Chromosome Number	Clinical condition
XX/XXY	46/47	Klinefelter's syndrome
XX/XO	46/45	Turner's syndrome
XO/XXX	45/47	Turner's syndrome
XO/XYY	45/47	Female in appearance with abnormal gonads
XY/XO/XX	46/45/46	Male in appearance with abnormal gonads
XO/XX/XXX	45/46/47	Variable Turner's syndrome

mosaicism has been found in an infant with the '*Cri du chat*' syndrome. As the deficient B group chromosome associated with this syndrome forms a ring, cells carrying it can easily be recognised, rendering such a case well suited for study. The cytological analysis revealed that although every cell of the child had 46 chromosomes, only 2 per cent were normal, in the other 98 per cent the ring chromosome was present. The case raises an important question as to why the chromosomally abnormal cell line fared so much better during embryonic development than the cells with the normal chromosome pattern. At present no satisfactory answer can be given to this question.

Another instance of autosomal mosaicism was observed in a newborn female. She had three cell lines: one was normal (46 chromosomes); the other was also normal as regards the number, but one chromosome in the E group had a deletion; the third cell line had 47 chromosomes with trisomy of chromosome no. 16.

Individuals with chromosomal mosaicism show very great variation in the manifestation of the pathological syndromes associated with the particular anomaly. This is attributed to the different proportion of the normal and abnormal cell lines present in the tissues. The cytogenetic anomaly may be present in one tissue but not in the others. Even when several tissues are affected, the proportion of 'mosaic' cells can be different among them. The variation of syndromes in similar chromosome mosaics is unpredictable. The abnormal types of XO/XY sex chromosome mosaics range from female with the features of Turner's syndrome to predominantly male; the relative proportion of cells is important but is not the only factor which determines the final outcome. It was found that the degree of mosaicism is not always correlated with the severity of Down's syndrome in mosaic mongols. The relative scarcity of mosaicism in which structurally altered chromosomes are involved seems to suggest that without a compensating change in the number of chromosomes, cells with gross structural chromosome change are non-viable.

The likelihood of detecting chromosome mosaicism depends on the tissue of origin in relation to development, on the extent of cell migration and on the rate of proliferation of the different cell types. When the ovarian tissue is chromosomally mosaic, the chromosome anomaly can be transmitted to the offspring through the egg. Such a case is on record. A woman who had two cell lines, one which was normal, the other which had 47 chromosomes with trisomy of chromosome no. 21., gave birth to mongol children!

The spontaneously aborted foetuses represent favourable material to study the types of chromosome anomalies, their distribution in the tissues and to correlate them with the severity of the developmental defects. Many such studies have been carried out, and they show that many of the foetuses which aborted in late pregnancy are chromosomal mosaics.

In view of the findings that chromosome anomalies occur at any stage of foetal development, it may be assumed that mitotic disturbances continue to occur in the *adult organism*, resulting in chromosomally abnormal cells. Such cells, however, could only be detected if the change took place in a cell which is proliferating and which provides a large number of descendant cells. This is the reason why cytologists looked for the possible presence of such cells in the haematopoietic tissue and cancerous growth.

Studies carried out since 1961 by W. M. Court Brown and his group in Edinburgh, revealed the absence of sex chromosomes in some of the blood cells of old persons. In males who were more than 65 years of age, cells have been found with 45 chromosomes, and the missing chromosome has been identified as the Y. A similar observation was made in females who were over 70 years of age; in these, one of the Xes was absent. The proportion of XO cells in males is 1·7 per cent, in females it is 7·3 per cent; these frequencies are significantly higher in old persons than in younger ones. Court Brown suggests that the loss of sex chromosomes may be associated with the hormonal changes which take place in persons of advanced age.

The findings of the Edinburgh group of cytologists were based on blood cells taken from individuals representing a cross-section of the general population. The arrival of the whole population of the island Tristan da Cunha in Great Britain in 1961 made possible the analysis of the chromosomes of a small, well isolated human population. J. L. Hamerton and his co-workers at Guy's Hospital, London, examined 78 per cent of the islanders and their results were similar to those obtained by the Edinburgh group. They also found that the number of aneuploid cells increases with increasing age. Hamerton suggested that the mechanism might be a general lowering of mitotic efficiency leading to loss of chromosomes. The chromosome imbalance results in the death of cells, and only those in which the missing chromosome is the X or Y can escape this fate.

The findings of the two groups of investigators can be considered to be a special case of chromosomal mosaicism in which the anomalous cell line arises late in life. Most commonly, the 'new' cell line originates early during foetal life and its cells can be recognised by the chromosomal changes present. Instances are known, however, in which the new cell line owes its origin to gene mutation and the cells do not display visible chromosome anomalies. In this connection, it is appropriate to draw attention to a situation which has peculiar features.

The situation is called '*chimaerism*', to distinguish it from mosaicism. In the latter the 'new' line is derived from a cell of the individual itself, in the former the 'new' line is derived from a different individual. The organism containing cells which have been derived, or obtained, from another genetically different individual is named chimaera after the mythical monster described by Homer, which had the head of a lion, the body of a goat and the tail of a serpent.

Chimaerism was first detected by the presence of two kinds of red blood cells in dizygotic (fraternal) twin cattle; the cells had evidently passed from one foetus to another through blood vessel linkages. In 1953 J. Dunsford and his associates reported the first case of blood cell chimaerism in man. A woman had a mixture of type A and O red cells; she was O, the other type was that of her twin brother. Since then, many similar instances of blood cell chimaerism have been described.

Blood cell chimaerism has also been induced by bone marrow transplantation. One such case is illustrated in Fig. 35.

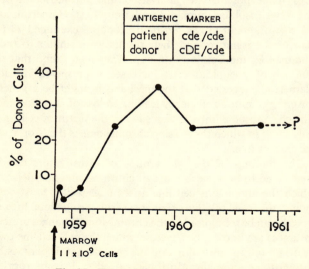

Fig. 35. *Human bone marrow chimaera; the donor cells could be recognised by the antigenic marker.*

The patient was intensively treated with a drug for her malignant condition and, as a consequence, the bone marrow was severely damaged. As a therapy, transfusion of marrow cells taken from a sister (non-twin) was administered to her, which resulted in the establishment of a new type of red cells of donor origin. The sister's donated red cells persisted for over two years in the recipient. The long survival of donor cells shows that the recipient patient developed a form of tolerance towards the foreign cells. The lack of response against these cells may be attributed to the impairment of the immune mechanism which is known to be associated with Hodgkin's disease, the malignant condition of the patient. Successful transplantation of tissues or organs (e.g. cornea, kidney) from donors to genetically different recipients can also be considered as another instance of chimaerism.

Another type of chimaerism has been produced by fusing together *in vitro* blastomeres from two or more genetically different embryos of mice into one composite group and transferring it into the uterus of pseudopregnant females. Dr Beatrice Mintz at the Institute for Cancer Research in Philadelphia obtained about 500 mice by this procedure, each animal being of multi-embryo origin, composed of genetically different tissues which show their particular characteristics. These mice are called *allophenic* because they display different genetic features in different regions of the body. When the embryos were fused, the immune mechanism was still nonexistent and the different components developed mutual tolerance, as revealed by skin grafting in the adult mice.

CHROMOSOME ANOMALIES AND CANCER

Cancer is a disease due to malignant growth which is the result of uncontrolled multiplication of tissue cells. The fact that cancerous or malignant tissue contains cells with an abnormal chromosome constitution was already known to the pathologists of the last century. The term 'chromosome' was just one year old when in 1889 Klebs described aberrant division of cells in tumour tissue and noted that in some cells the number of chromosome bodies is very large. The earliest systematic study of cell division in human tumours was carried out by von Hansemann. In several reports published between 1890 and 1906 he described in detail the various mitotic anomalies seen in tumours, and attributed the unusually large or small number of chromosomes to the formation of an abnormal spindle (Plates XIV & XV). Hansemann argued that the irregular distribution of chromosomes disturbs the balance between nucleus and cytoplasm, and suggested that the discordance between them is the cause of malignant behaviour of cells.

Hansemann's idea was carried further by T. Boveri. His experiments with sea urchins convinced him that for normal development and tissue organisation a definite chromosome constitution is essential. Boveri found that in sea-urchin eggs fertilised with two sperms, multipolar spindles are formed, causing unequal distribution of chromosomes in the daughter cells. Furthermore, he observed that the cells thus produced failed to arrange themselves into the regular tissue pattern and that the cell aggregate resembled cancerous tissue. These findings led Boveri to put forward a theory in 1912 according to which malignant growth originates in cells which acquired an abnormal chromosome content. This view, though it was held by one of the best embryologists, was not accepted at the time. Owing to the difficulties of preparing animal tissues for chromosome studies, no crucial evidence could be obtained to confirm Boveri's findings.

Since 1956, when improved cytological techniques became available, a great body of observation has been collected by analysing the chromosome constitution of cells in experimentally induced and transplanted animal tumours. It was soon established that the chromosome constitution of the tumour cells was different from that of normal cells. It was also found that the chromosome pattern varied within the same tumour and between different tumours and that it was neither uniform nor stable. Some chromosome variants are more numerous than others, the largest class is referred to as the 'stem-line', containing the most favoured cells which are assumed responsible for the growth of the tumour. The cell populations of animal tumours provide an example of extreme chromosomal mosaicism.

The cytological studies of human tumours yielded similar results to those obtained from animal tumours. The large number of reports which have been published describe a wide spectrum of numerical and structural changes in the chromosomes of tumour cells. The conclusion which could be drawn from these studies was indefinite, vague and discouraging. The discovery of trisomy of chromosome no. 21 as the cause of a pathological state in man (mongolism) gave a new impetus to the study of human tumours in the expectation of finding evidence of a chromosomal basis of malignancy. The first important observation came from Philadelphia. P. C. Nowell and D. A. Hungerford reported in 1960 that an abnormal chromosome no. 21 is associated with chronic myeloid leukaemia. Their finding was soon corroborated by other cytologists. The faulty chromosome, referred to as the Philadelphia, or Ph′, chromosome, is shorter than its normal partner due to the loss of about two-thirds of the long arm (Plate IX *above*). Much discussion has been devoted to the Ph′ chromosome by cytologists and clinicians as to whether the deletion is the cause of the malignant disease. This question is, however, still under debate; at present we can state that the true importance of the Philadelphia chromosome lies in the fact that it is the first instance in which a specific chromosomal change became a characteristic feature of a particular malignant condition.

Whether cancerous behaviour of cells has a chromosomal basis or not can only be decided by identifying the cell which is in the actual process of malignant transformation and by studying the chromosomes. While such an investigation *in vivo* is out of the question, it became possible by following the events occurring within cells infected *in vitro* with tumour-producing viruses such as the polyoma virus in rodents. When embryonic cells of hamsters grown in cultures are infected with polyoma virus, the colonies of the infected cells exhibit numerous chromosomal anomalies, and some of these colonies develop tumours when transplanted back into adults. It seems that the virus-initiated transformation involves in some manner the DNA of the host cell causing chromosome anomalies. The chromosomal alterations can produce a metabolic state in the cytoplasm which may facilitate or even predispose the cell towards a malignant change.

The finding of J. Vinograd at the California Institute of Technology suggests that a particular cytoplasmic component of the cell may be involved in the process of carcinogenesis. He discovered a new type of DNA shaped in a series of rings, connected like links in a chain. It was found in the mitochondria of HeLa cells derived from carcinoma of the cervix and grown *in vitro* since 1952, and in the while blood cells of leukaemic patients. As the cancer viruses (e.g. polyoma, SV-40) have circular DNA, the question that arises is whether the new complex mitrochondrial DNA is a virus which is responsible for the cancerous behaviour of the cell. Further investigation revealed a correspondence between the various types of complex DNA and the behaviour of cancer cells. It was found that the relative amounts of mitochondrial DNA present as interlocked rings and single rings vary with the degree of advancement of the malignant condition. HeLa cells, derived from advanced cancer, contain almost exclusively interlocked rings of mitochondrial DNA; the pattern is similar in the white cells of advanced leukaemia patients, while in the early stages of leukaemia the cells contain mostly unlinked rings of mitochondrial DNA.

The best example that cells with chromosomal changes are more prone to become tumour cells is provided by studying the chromosome behaviour of cells grown *in vitro* for a considerable length of time. Culturing foetal skin cells of mice, A. Levan and J. Biesele observed a progressive alteration in the chromosome constitution. After the seventh passage it was found that the cells became *heteroploid*, i.e. they showed great variation in the number of chromosomes. When the cultured cells were transplanted into mice, they multiplied and developed into tumours. Another kind of evidence that the presence of a chromosome anomaly may predispose to cancer comes from Christchurch, New Zealand. F. W. Gunz and his associates found a family, several members of which had an

abnormal chromosome no. 21, in this instance the short arm
of the chromosome (referred to as Ch′) was deleted (Plate X).
The deficient chromosome appears to be associated with
lymphocytic leukaemia (Fig. 36).

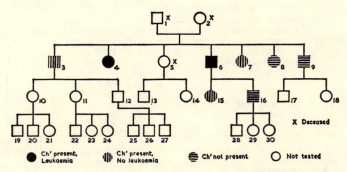

Fig. 36. *Pedigree of C-family, showing the possible association of the abnormal Ch′ chromosome with leukaemia.*

It has been reported that mongolism due to trisomy of
chromosome no. 21 is associated with a lymphocytic type of
leukaemia. A survey by Dr Alice Stewart shows that the
incidence is 20 times higher in mongol children than in the
general population. Recent studies revealed that other
pathological conditions due to, or associated with, chromosome anomalies (e.g. Klinefelter's, Turner's syndromes) have
a high frequency of cancer.

The most interesting examples of association between a
hereditary disease and cancer are provided by Fanconi's
anaemia and Bloom's syndrome. Both conditions are caused
by an autosomal recessive gene and are characterised by a
high frequency of cells with chromosome anomalies and an
increased tendency to cancer. It may be argued that the
chromosome anomaly is the manifestation of cellular instability due to the gene. Cellular instability in Fanconi's
syndrome has been demonstrated by culturing skin cells of
patients and by infecting them with the tumour-producing
Simian virus (SV–40), and noting the number of cells

'transformed'. The morphological features and the growth pattern of cell colonies derived from transformed cells are very pronounced and can easily be recognised. Table 17 shows

Table 17. *Frequency of cell transformation* in vitro *by SV–40.**

Source of cells	Number of transformed colonies†
Controls (7)	1·6–5·1
Fanconi's anaemia	
Homozygotes:	
AM	79·7 ± 18·1
JV	41·1 ± 12·1
Heterozygotes:	
TM	20·1 ± 3·2
CV	28·2 ± 8·7

* When injected into newborn hamsters, tumours are produced in the adult animals.

† 10 000 cells plated.

that the cells from patients with Fanconi's syndrome transform at least 50 times more frequently than cells from normal persons.

The association observed between chromosome anomalies and predisposition to cancer suggests that chromosomal disturbance could be one of the signals of the abnormal cellular condition which is part of the 'cancerisation' process of cells. It might be possible to use chromosome aberrations occurring in the cells of persons who are exposed to various environmental agents as indicators of their carcinogenic hazards. Chromosome studies of workers exposed to benzene, a known inducer of leukaemia, have already been made, and the incidence of chromosome anomalies was found to be nearly three times higher in them than in non-exposed persons. The Edinburgh group of cytogeneticists recently reported a high frequency and long survival of chromosome anomalies in patients who have been exposed to Thorotrast, a colloidal suspension containing the radioactive thorium-232. This substance is used as a control medium for X-ray diagnosis of pathological lesions in particular tissues. When injected intravenously it is deposited in the spleen, liver and bone marrow, exposing the cells to continuous radiation by α-particles. It was discovered in 1956 that Thorotrast produces leukaemia, and since then its use has been discontinued. The cytological analysis of persons who underwent this diagnostic method 11–37 years previously has revealed that 9·2 per cent of their blood cells had chromosome anomalies, and that nearly 6 per cent of these were stable and could survive indefinitely

A similar finding is reported concerning some of the Marshall Islanders who were exposed to radioactive fall-out in 1954. Fourteen years later it was found that 23 out of 43 persons examined had chromosome abnormalities of the stable type. Some of the Islanders have already developed leukaemia.

Recently, several reports were published describing chromosome anomalies in persons who have suffered viral infections, or undergone various drug treatments. One report concerns LSD (lysergic acid diethylamide) used for the treatment of paranoid schizophrenia by psychiatrists, which is suspected to be a possible agent inducing chromosome anomalies. This drug is being misused by young people, without their realising the possible danger involved. No doubt only time will show how high the carcinogenic hazard is of this and other chemical agents to which man is now exposed.

Though the above findings are very suggestive in establishing a causal association between chromosome anomaly and cancer, they cannot be construed as evidence to confirm Boveri's theory. According to him, chromosome irregularity is the direct cause of malignant cell behaviour. It is now known from biological and biochemical studies that carcinogenesis is a complex phenomenon in which chromosome disturbance – if it occurs at all – is only a part of the whole process. The gross chromosomal abnormalities seen in already established tumours are secondary phenomena which occur in an apparently haphazard fashion. Recent studies indicate, however, that the extensive alterations in chromosome number and structure may represent definite stages in the evolution of new karyotypes.

Evidence is slowly accumulating that similar 'marker chromosomes', i.e. chromosomes which have undergone structural alteration, are present in similar tumours (Plate XVI). The studies of chromosomes in tumours are providing a continuous flow of information which may eventually help the clinicians to diagnose precancerous lesions, to estimate the degree of malignancy of tumours and their response to treatment.

The chromosomally heterogeneous cell composition observed in cancerous growths of plants and animals, including man, represents a special kind of mosaicism in adult organisms.

5. The Genetic Load and Future of Man

Evolution of a species, including man, is the result of mutation. The genetic differences between individuals are the raw material on which natural selection acts. The hereditary mechanism is responsible for recombining the mutations into variable patterns, from which natural selection chooses the individuals who best fit and adapt to a given environment. Mutations provide variability, and for this reason, they are necessary for evolutionary progress. Extensive studies have, however, demonstrated the fact that the greatest proportion of mutations are deleterious to the individual who carries the mutated gene. It was found in experiments that, for every successful or useful mutation, there are many thousands which are harmful. Swedish plant breeders produced a variety of barley with a high yield by irradiating the seeds, but they had to discard a vast number of inferior mutants which had arisen together with the rare superior ones.

Genetic variants of low fitness are continuously arising in all living species, and several generations may elapse before such mutations are eliminated. Beside the inherited deleterious mutations, frequently a new harmful mutation is added to the genetic burden. The sum total of such genes comprises the 'genetic load', which is a serious burden not only to the individual, but also to the population, race and species.

The number of those genes which affect only the 'fitness' of individuals is also believed to be increasing. Fitness may be defined as a genetically determined adaptation of an individual to a given environmental condition. Reduction in fitness is reflected in shorter life-span, predisposition to disease, lowered intelligence, etc. Geneticists have demonstrated that recessive genes of Drosophila, even in the heterozygous individuals which do not show the mutations, have some deleterious, measurable effects on 'fitness'. The higher the number of such genes, the greater the adverse effect on the fitness of the individual. We humans are loaded with such genes.

H. J. Muller studied the implication of the genetic burden on the future of man. According to him, one person in five is born with a detrimental gene derived from mutation in the germ cells of his or her parents, in addition to those which have been accumulated and handed down from earlier ancestors. The hidden store of deleterious genes is revealed by consanguineous marriages, since the genetic constitutions of close relatives are similar. The incidence of still-birth and diseased offspring is much higher in marriages between first cousins than in the general population. According to the 1964 report issued by the World Health Organisation, the death rate of children whose parents are 'blood relations' is nearly four times higher than of those born to parents not related to one another. A report from Japan on the fate of seven children of a marriage between first cousins illustrated the serious consequences of the hidden deleterious genes: one child was still-born, three lived only a few days, one died from acute leukaemia at the age of three months, and two survived for several years at the time of observation. Dr C. O. Carter of the Clinical Genetics Research Unit, London, reported on 13 incestuous children born in 1958–59 from six father–daughter and seven brother–sister marriages. When the position was reviewed in 1965, three of the children had died of hereditary conditions, one child was severely subnormal, four educationally subnormal, and only five were found to be more or less normal. These are a few examples to indicate the existence of the hidden store of deleterious mutations present in human populations. Muller estimates that about six per cent of all persons are born with some tangible loss of fitness due to gene mutations. It is therefore not surprising for some biologists to believe that while our cultural and technical evolution progresses, biologically mankind is degenerating rather than improving.

The frequency of some *dominant* gene mutations in man has been estimated. When the genetic defect is very severe, and the reproductive fitness of the individual is low, it can be assumed that the appearance of a similar genetic defect is due to a *new* mutation in the same gene. The occurrence of chondrodystrophic dwarfism (adult body proportions with short arms and legs) has been studied in Denmark. Eight such dwarfs were found amongst 94 075 children born in a Copenhagen hospital. On this data it is estimated that the rate of mutation is 1 in 12 000 births. Pelger anomaly, which affects the white cells in the blood and is associated with a reduced resistance to disease, occurs with nearly the same frequency. In Britain every year about 36 haemophilic children are born, victims of a new mutation in the sex-linked gene of haemophilia.

The mutation rate for *recessive* traits like albinism or phenylketonuria is more difficult to estimate for various reasons, one of the most important being that the proportion of heterozygotes in the human population is continuously

Table 18. *Estimated rates of mutations in man.*

Mutation	Effect	Frequency once in *n* gametes
DOMINANT		
Pelger anomaly	Abnormal white blood cells	12 500
Chondrodystrophic dwarfism	Shortened limbs	12 000
Retinoblastoma	Tumours on the retina	43 500
Epiloia	Tumour in brain	83 000–120 000
RECESSIVE		
Haemophilia	Failure of blood clotting	32 000
Colour-blindness (total)	Failure to distinguish colours	36 000
Albinism	Lack of melanin	36 000

increasing due to medical care and social welfare. Some estimated rates of mutations in man are given in Table 18.

So far we have considered 'spontaneous' gene mutations of deleterious traits as the source of the genetic burden in man.

The frequency of gene mutations can, however, be increased by environmental agents, amongst which ionising radiations (X-rays, gamma and neutron radiation) are the most powerful. The somatic effects of X-rays are well known; individuals exposed to excessive amounts suffer injuries resulting in cancer and death. The mutagenic effect of radiation on the gene was discovered by H. J. Muller in 1927. The mutations obtained from this external agent are the same as those arising spontaneously, but they are more frequent.

Fig. 37 illustrates the proportion of the various types of mutations as observed by Muller in 1000 offspring of male flies

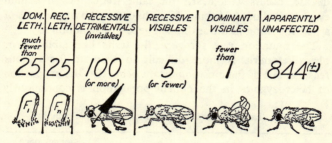

Fig. 37. *Schematic representation of the effects estimated by H. J. Muller to be produced by 1000 rads in 1000 offspring of irradiated male flies.*

irradiated with 1000 rads. The visible mutations are weaker, less fertile, and shorter-lived than normal flies; other mutations reduce vigour, longevity and fertility without altering the appearance of the flies. These effects on fitness could only be detected by laborious tests devised by Muller himself.

The most important finding was that the effects produced by radiation are *directly* proportional to the amount of radiation received. Three per cent of the sperms carry a new radiation-induced mutation when the fly is exposed to 1000 rads; this proportion is increased to six and nine per cent when the dose is increased to 2000 rads and 3000 rads respectively. These results led Muller to conclude that the frequency of mutations depends on the magnitude of the radiation dose.

It was also discovered that the way of administering the dose did not affect the mutation rate; 1000 rads given in 30 minutes or given in 30 days produced an equal number of gene mutations. This finding is of extreme importance to man, who is exposed more often to small amounts of radiation than to large doses. Furthermore, it is immaterial whether the dose, e.g. 25 rads, is distributed amongst 25 or 2500 people, the number of mutations produced is the same!

In addition to producing gene mutation, radiation also produces chromosome injuries; deletion, inversion and translocation, all of which have genetic consequences previously discussed (Plate XII *below*). Some of the chromosome anomalies may persist for several months or years after exposure. Dividing cells with chromosome aberrations have been found in a worker who was exposed 20 years previously to radiation during an accident at an Atomic Energy Establishment. Studies carried out by the Edinburgh group of cytogeneticists have shown that the frequency of chromosome aberrations is higher in personnel engaged in occupations where they are exposed to the hazards of ionising radiation as compared with the general population.

In view of the ever-increasing use of radiation in medicine and industry, an International Committee has advised that 5 rads per year is the permissible dose to which any individual may be exposed. In setting the annual dose at 5 rads, the Committee was trying to balance the benefit by applying radiation in medicine and industry and the possible genetic hazards.

Since the discovery by C. Auerbach of the mutagenic effect of mustard gas, many more chemical mutagens have been reported, based mostly on experimental data obtained with Drosophila, Neurospora and bacteria. Some of these mutagens are listed in Table 19. This table also indicates the source of those chemicals to which man might be exposed. Whether these agents penetrate as effective mutagens into the germ cells of man is, however, still uncertain. It should also be emphasised that the action of a chemical mutagen depends on its absorption, distribution and diffusion through the tissues and cells. In spite of these difficulties, serious consideration should be given to the possibility that the number of deleterious mutations in man can be increased by chemical contaminants of our environment.

Table 19. *Some effective chemical mutagens.*

	Droso-phila	Neuro-spora	Bacteria	Source of exposure
Mustard derivatives (Chlorambucil)	+	+	+	Cancer therapy
Epoxides	+	+	+	Industry and domestic use
Imines	+	+	+	Cancer therapy
Alkane-sulphonic esters (Myleran)	+	+	+	Cancer therapy
Peroxides	+	+	+	Smog
Aldehydes	+	+	+	Industry Disinfectant
Purines (Caffeine)	±	?	+	Beverages

Another way by which the genetic load of man is increasing is due to our own actions. We have created conditions in which the survival not only of the fittest but also of many physically debilitated and mentally defective is assured. Such individuals are sheltered by medicine and social welfare; they can survive and can disseminate their inferior genetic make-up into the population. Forty years ago a diabetic patient would have died before marriageable age; today, under medical care, he lives long enough to have children and through them preserves his deleterious gene.

Two problems are facing the biologist of today: (i) how to alleviate genetic disease and (ii) how to better man genetically. As regards the first, several methods can be applied and are in use, which make life more tolerable for the carriers of genetic defects. Thus by eliminating phenylalanine from the diet very early in life, one prevents the irreversible damage the child could have expected when born with phenylketonuria (PKU). The incidence of PKU is 1 in 10 000 births. A simple method, devised in 1960, is now in use for screening large numbers of infants. In the United States, since 1965, 32 States have passed the 'PKU laws' instructing pediatricians to do such screening. The legislation went through mainly on account of saving the institutional expenses for PKU-retarded children. Diets low in phenylalanine are now prescribed as treatment. According to recent reports, many PKU women on such diets have produced mentally retarded children. Some pediatricians believe that the dietary therapy may affect the foetus during pregnancy, causing mental retardation.

When the genetic disease is due to the lack of a gene product, this may be replaced. Such a disease is haemophilia, where the enzyme necessary for blood clotting is missing. The carrier of this condition can be greatly helped by administering anti-haemolytic globulin, which promotes the clotting of blood.

Spina bifida is another serious genetic disease to which modern surgical intervention has brought great improvements. The child afflicted with this condition is born with the spinal cord exposed, resulting in paralysis of the lower half of the body with lack of control of bowels and bladder, and in many cases the disease is associated with hydrocephaly (water on the brain). In this country each year about 900 children are born with spina bifida. Once a child with spina bifida is born to a family there is a 1 in 40 chance that subsequent children will also be affected. A few years ago four out of five cases proved fatal but now surgical closure of the spine saves half of the victims, and special facilities are being provided by the Education Authorities to overcome the disabilities of such children, with some success.

These methods of treatment, while of great value to individual patients, have no *genetic* value for the human race. In treating and not curing the cause of the disease, the deleterious genes are preserved.

The question as to the wisdom of allowing genetically handicapped people to reproduce leads us to discuss the second problem, how to better the human race. In about 1800, Galton initiated the 'Eugenics' movement. Its aim was to improve the human race by preventing reproduction of the genetically unfit and by the selective breeding of desirable types. Two serious criticisms have been levelled against the aim of eugenics, which is based upon arbitrary valuations of individuals and social groups. First, in certain environments a 'bad gene' may be an advantage. This is well illustrated in the case of sickle-cell anaemia, as the gene confers an advantage on the carrier, who is more resistant than normal people are to malaria. Secondly, who should decide what is the 'desirable' type to be chosen for selective breeding, and how? What sort of man is the ideal to be striven for?

The subject of genetic improvement of man has been discussed recently at a symposium organised by the CIBA Foundation in London. The Nobel laureate Muller argued with 'evangelical zeal' for 'genetic progress by voluntarily conducted germinal choice', recommending artificial insemination. The sperms would be collected from selected donors, with 'superior germ plasm', outstanding either physically or intellectually. The sperms would be stored in sperm banks and utilised according to demands. The programme outlined by Muller met much criticism by biologists who do not accept his pessimistic view. The chief questions are: who will be the President of the National Sperm Bank, and who will guard the National DNA Bank? According to Th. Dobzhansky, Professor of Biology and Genetics at the Rockefeller Institute, New York, modern evolutionary biology justifies a more optimistic view of man's biological future than that expressed by Muller.

With the new knowledge of the gene, its organisation and function, geneticists are speculating on other methods by which our genetic load may be lightened. One of the visionaries is J. Lederberg of Stanford University, California, who advocates *'euphenics'*, the engineering of human development, in an aim to compensate for certain genetic defects. According to Lederberg, the medical revolution of today may lead us to invent new techniques, e.g. synthesis of hormones, enzymes, antigens and proteins. It may also be possible to design gene programmed reactions. Lederberg believes that further discoveries in molecular genetics may permit us to practise '*algeny*', i.e. to alter genes in the body cells or in the germinal tissues, or to introduce the desired genes from outside. Phenylketonuria might be cured by infecting the infant who has the disease with a 'silent' virus, which can code for the missing enzyme phenylalanine hydroxylase without producing pathological aberrations. A 'silent' virus in man has recently been identified by S. Rodgers at the Oak Ridge National Laboratories in the United States; it is the Shope virus which in rabbits produces skin papilloma and tumours. Its presence in humans who became infected was revealed by the alteration of the enzyme arginase, which is common in the human cell. No other effects have been seen in the human host carrying the Shope virus.

One of the most novel ideas, which has been put forward by Lederberg, is the application of vegetative or asexual propagation to man. By this method, which is practised very effectively by horticulturalists, genetically uniform colonies of plants can be grown and propagated. Lederberg argues that instead of trying to modify a genetic anomaly by reprogramming the DNA either in the reproductive cells or in every somatic cell, methods are now available which could enable us to practise 'clonal reproduction'. This process would require the transfer of somatic cell nuclei into the fertilised and enucleated egg (similar to the procedure employed by Volpe and McKinnel to produce clones of frogs; see p. 31). According to Lederberg, the dormant storage of human germ plasm as sperm could be replaced by freezing somatic tissues to save potential donor nuclei, chosen for their 'superior' or 'desirable' genetic constitution.

These are 'alluring vistas', no doubt encouraged by the very discoveries which we discussed in this book. The time is not yet here when we can practise the art of switching on at will the desirable genes and switching off the undesirable ones. There are still vast areas of ignorance to be converted into precise knowledge before we can practise 'genetic surgery' and embark on controlling human heredity and evolution.

Man of today is the heir of all ages, he is the product of many millions of years of hard-won evolution. It is the duty, not only of biologists but of all mankind, to safeguard the genetic heritage by minimising the dangers which may arise from the world around us. The information presented here should help readers to understand the reasons for our obligations.

Appendix to the 1971 Edition

Since the publication of this book, some important discoveries have been made to which the author feels the reader's attention should be drawn.

(i) *Kornberg's enzyme: DNA-polymerase* (p. 28)

For the *in vitro* (test-tube) synthesis of DNA of the Coli bacterium, a particular enzyme is required and is produced by the gene 'DNA-polymerase', which represents only a very small portion of the cell DNA. Extensive and careful experiments carried out by Cairns and co-workers in 1969 showed, however, that this enzyme is used for the repair of DNA rather than for its replication. They were able to demonstrate this fact by using a mutant type of Coli bacteria, in which the greatest part of the 'DNA-polymerase' gene was deleted, so that these mutants contained less than one percent of the polymerase activity present in the wild type cells; yet they found that the DNA strands of the mutants were still able to duplicate. Thus the binding together of the indvidual nucleotide bases must be attributed to another enzyme, the search for which was still in progress in 1970. Cairns suggests that Kornberg's polymerase is a 'repair' enzyme, whose function is to obliterate any faulty regions in the DNA duplex which may arise during replication, and to restore the correct sequence of nucleotide base pairing. Thus the role of the Kornberg enzyme is that of editing rather than assisting in the process of actual DNA double helix duplication.

(ii) *The 'Central Dogma' of Crick* (p. 83)

It has been firmly established that the amino acid composition of proteins is coded in DNA, and is specified by the sequence of nucleotide bases. According to Crick, 'once the sequential information has passed from DNA to RNA and into protein, it cannot get out again'; his statement has been referred to as the

'Central Dogma.' The validity of this generalisation has been questioned recently because of experimental work by Temin and Baltimore. These workers were able to provide evidence that RNA can sometimes serve as a template for complementary DNA, and thus the direction of passing information is RNA to DNA; Temin and Baltimore used tumour-producing viruses containing only RNA as the source of genetic information, and found that when such RNA tumour viruses infect cells, they produce DNA characteristic of the virus and not of the infected cells. They concluded that the transfer of genetic information from RNA to DNA is possible. This finding, supported by other research workers, led to some scientists' suggesting that the 'Central Dogma' is an oversimplification. Crick, in his defence, argues that his original statement did not rule out the transfer of genetic information from RNA to DNA and then by the normal process to RNA and protein (RNA to DNA to RNA to protein), but he upheld the conviction that it is not possible to convert the genetic information contained in protein molecules back into the genetic information embodied in DNA (protein to DNA). This is the true essence of the 'Central Dogma' according to Crick.

If a cell system were found which could carry out transfers from protein to DNA, it would shake the very foundation of molecular biology. There is, however, still the possibility that in the primaeval conditions in which the first living things emerged, protein molecules may have been the sources of genetic information, and our present system in which continuity of living organisms is dependent on nucleic acid molecules evolved subsequently.

(iii) Khorana's synthetic gene (p. 135)

In view of the great advances made in the field of molecular biology, scientists considering the genetic basis of many diseases in man expressed the hope that it might be possible to provide the normal gene to tissues of affected individuals. This possibility came nearer to reality with the discovery made by H. G. Khorana at the Institute of Enzyme Research in Wisconsin. He may be considered to be the first to accomplish the *in vitro* synthesis of a gene responsible for the alanine-transfer RNA enzyme in yeast. The chemical composition of this rather simple enzyme was clarified by R. Holley at the Salk Institute of California, and it thus became possible to deduce the structure of the gene coding for this enzyme from the sequence of the amino acids in the polypeptide chain. Khorana joined together the four nucleotides (adenine, thymine, cysteine and guanine) step by step to form short single stranded segments. Then using the enzyme 'DNA-ligase' extracted and purified from living cells, these were linked into the double-stranded DNA-gene consisting of 77 nucleotide bases. This 'artificial' gene was introduced into a mutant yeast in which the gene coding for the alanine-transfer RNA enzyme was absent, and the mutant yeast was transformed into a normal yeast. Khorana's achievement is of great significance, since he worked out the rules for gene synthesis, and it seems that theoretically any desired gene could be manufactured in test tubes in the future.

(iv) *AUG triplet; the initiator of protein synthesis* (p. 82)

Since the 'cracking of the genetic code', molecular biologists have been investigating the problem of how the ribosome is instructed to translate the information from mRNA to produce the polypeptide chain of a particular protein. It now seems that the research has succeeded, revealing that the triplet AUG is the initiator of the process. This triplet codes for the amino acid methionine, but special structural arrangements of the mRNA make it possible for the ribosome to discriminate between using the AUG as an initiator or simply as a code for incorporating methionine as one amino acid component of a polypeptide chain. It was found that the mRNA produced by phages folds up into a number of hairpin-like loops, and that at the top of each loop is found the AUG triplet. It was assumed that this instructs the ribosome to commence the translation of the message into protein synthesis. The essential feature of this arrangement is that although there are many AUG triplets along the mRNA it is only those which are exposed at the tip of the loop which can act as initiators. Holley at the Massachusetts Institute of Technology provided evidence that during breakage of these mRNA loops more AUG triplets were exposed, and as a consequence could act as triplet-initiators, the ribosome thus producing more protein than it normally would. This has been found to occur in the synthesis of haemoglobin in the reticulocytes of rabbit, and also in protamine synthesis in the sperms of trout. It is therefore assumed that the amino acid methionine is the "universal initiator" for protein synthesis, a concept which is now becoming widely accepted amongst molecular biologists.

Appendices

APPENDIX I. DIMENSIONS IN MILLIMETRES (mm), MICRONS (μ) AND ÅNGSTROMS (Å)

$$
\begin{array}{lll}
1\cdot 0 \text{ mm} & = & 1000\ \mu \\
0\cdot 1 \text{ mm} & = & 100\ \mu \\
10^{-2}\text{mm} & = & 10\ \mu \\
10^{-3}\text{mm} & = & 1\ \mu \\
10^{-4}\text{mm} & = & 0\cdot 1\ \mu & = 1000 \text{ Å} \\
10^{-5}\text{mm} & = & 0\cdot 01\ \mu & = 100 \text{ Å} \\
10^{-6}\text{mm} & = & 0\cdot 001\ \mu & = 10 \text{ Å} \\
10^{-7}\text{mm} & = & 0\cdot 0001\mu & = 1 \text{ Å}
\end{array}
$$

Cells
Bacteria
Viruses
Proteins
Amino acids

* Limit of resolution by light microscope.
† Limit of resolution by electron microscope.

APPENDIX II. NOBEL PRIZES IN PHYSIOLOGY AND MEDICINE
AWARDED TO SCIENTISTS IN THE FIELD OF GENETICS

Year	Scientists	Nature of work
1934	Thomas Hunt Morgan	Research leading to a new concept of the gene, the basic unit of heredity
1946	Herman J. Muller	The induction of gene mutations by X-rays
1958	George W. Beadle Edward L. Tatum Joshua Lederberg	Fundamental discoveries in the field of biochemical and bacterial genetics
1959	Arthur Kornberg Severo Ochoa	Research on the chemistry of DNA and RNA and on their relationship
1961	James D. Watson Francis H. C. Crick Maurice H. F. Wilkins	Investigation into the molecular structure of DNA leading to the discovery of the Genetic Code

Bibliography

AUERBACH, C. *Genetics in the Atomic Age*, 2nd Edit. Oliver & Boyd
Edinburgh. 1965.
Semi-popular book explaining clearly the genetic consequences
of radiation.

BEADLE, G. and BEADLE, MURIEL. 1966. *The Language of Life*.
Gollancz, London.
A semi-popular introduction to 'molecular genetics' by a
Nobel Prize winner and his wife; the book has many interesting
historical references.

CARLSON, E. 1966. *The Gene: A Critical History*. W. B. Saunders,
Philadelphia.
Describes the work of the Morgan school, how the discoveries
were made and to whom the credit is due.

DARLINGTON, C. D. 1958. *Evolution of Genetic Systems*, 2nd Edit.
Oliver & Boyd, Edinburgh.
Excellent description of the role chromosomes played in
evolution, written by the founder of cytogenetics.

SRB, A. M., OWEN, R. D. and EDGAR, R. S. 1965. *General Genetics*,
2nd Edit. W. F. Freeman, San Francisco and London.
An exhaustive textbook.

SULLIVAN, N. 1967. *The Message of the Genes*. Basic Books, New
York.
Historical review of recent discoveries relating to DNA.

THOMPSON, J. S. and THOMPSON, MARGARET. 1966. *Genetics and
Medicine*. W. B. Saunders, Philadelphia and London.
Clear presentation of all the basic knowledge of genetics, for
the use of medical students.

WATSON, J. D. 1962. *The Molecular Biology of the Gene*. Benjamin,
New York and Amsterdam.
Classical book by the Nobel laureate containing in detail the pro-
gress of DNA genetics.

WINCHESTER, A. M. 1964. *Heredity, an Introduction to Genetics*.
Harrap, London.
Textbook dealing briefly with all aspects of genetics, its methods
and applications.

Acknowledgements

I am grateful to Messrs W. B. Saunders and Co., Philadelphia, for permission to use some of their illustrations (Figs. 4, 8, 11 & 14); and to Messrs G. G. Harrap and Co., London, for Fig. 21. For providing me with photographs and diagrams, I wish to express my indebtedness to the following: Dr R. E. Billingham, University of Pennsylvania, Philadelphia (Fig. 23); Dr E. P. Volpe, Tulane University, New Orleans (Fig. 13); Drs F. W. Gunz and P. H. Fitzgerald, Royal Children's Hospital, Christchurch (Fig. 36, and Plates IX *below* & X); Dr J. Hamerton, Guy's Hospital, London (Plate VIII); Mr L. LaCour, John Innes Institute, Norwich (Plates II *above* & V); and to my colleagues, Drs Sylvia D. Lawler (Plate IX *above*), S. H. Revell (Plate XII), P. D. Lawley (Fig. 28), D. T. Hughes (Plates III, IV, VI & VII), and Mr M. S. C. Birbeck (Plate I). My thanks are also due to Mr E. A. Sykes for drawing some of the diagrams and to the Photographic Department, particularly Mr M. J. Docherty, for technical assistance. For the help given to me by my secretary, Miss Marjorie Butt, and by Mr D. A. Brunning for reading the proofs, I am most grateful.

I wish also to acknowledge the helpful advice received from Mr I. A. G. Le Bek, Editor of Contemporary Science Paperbacks, and to thank Miss O. M. Hamilton on his staff in particular.

P.C.K.

Index

ABO blood groups, 59–60, 61, 62
Abortion, 110, 111, 112
Acetabularia, 7, 8
Acridine, 92
Acrocentric, 22, 26
Adenine, 13, 14, 15, 16
Agglutination, 60, 61
Albinism, 74, 129
Aldehyde, 132
Algeny, 135
Alkane sulphonic ester, 132
Alkaptonuria, 74
Allele, 45
Allophenic, 119
ALS (antilymphocyte serum), 68
Amenorrhoea, 109
Amino acid, 2, 71, 72, 73, 74, 76
Amino purine, 92
Amoeba, 5, 6
Anaemia, 93, 123
Anaphase, 20
Aneuploidy, 100, 112
Antibody, 59
Antigen, 59, 63, 64
Asexual, 135
ATP (adenosine triphosphate), 4
Aulacantha, 23
Autograft, 65
Auto-immunity, 70
Autosome, 23
Azaserine, 92

Bacterial transformation, 10, 11
Barr body, 54

Benzene, 124
Blastula, 32
Bloom's syndrome, 123
Bromouracil, 93

Caffeine, 132
Cancer, 5, 69, 92, 119, 120, 121, 139
Centriole, 3, 4, 20
Centromere, 20, 21
Centrosome, 3
Chiasma, 35, 48
Chimaerism, 118–119
Chlorambucil, 132
Chlorophyll, 2
Chloroplast, 2, 4
Chondrodystrophy, 129
Chromatid, 20
Chromatin, 9
Chromocentre, 9
Chromosome, 18
Code, 80, 82
Co-dominant, 60
Codon, 80
Co-linearity, 78
Colour blindness, 50, 112, 129
Consanguineous marriage, 128
Contact inhibition, 5
Cri du chat syndrome, 110, 115
Crossing-over, 48, 101
Cross-linking, 92, 93
Cytogenetics, 97
Cytoplasm, 2
Cytosine, 13

Deletion, 100, 109, 131
Diabetes, 55, 132

Diploid (2*n*), 24
DNA (deoxyribonucleic acid),
    9, 13–18, 27, 29, 31, 83, 135
DNA polymerase, 28
DNA template, 28
Dominant, 38
Down's syndrome, 103, 105,
    109
Drosophila, 46, 47, 49, 50, 57,
    59, 71, 72, 90, 130
D-trisomy, 106
Duplication, 101, 109

Eczema, 70
Endoplasmic reticulum (ER),
    2, 4
Enzyme, 21, 72–74, 75, 85
Epiloia, 129
Epoxide, 132
Ergastoplasm, 2
Erythroblastosis foetalis, 62, 63
Escherichia coli (*E. coli*), 11,
    88, 89, 112
Esterases, 85
E-trisomy, 106
Eugenics, 133
Euphenics, 134

Fertilisation, 33
Feulgen reaction, 21
Fitness, 128
Fluorouracil, 92

Gamete, 24, 33, 39, 41, 43, 45
Gamma globulin, 64
Gastrula, 90
Gene, 46
Genetic code, 80–82
Genetic load, 127
Genetic map, 112
Genetics, 45
Genetic sex, 54
Genome, 83, 113
Germinal mutation, 95
Golgi body, 3, 4
Gout, 55

G-trisomy (Down's syndrome),
    103, 104
Guanine, 13
G6PD (enzyme), 52, 112

Haemoglobin, 75, 76, 85, 89
Haemophilia, 50, 51, 52, 112,
    129, 133
Haploid (*n*), 24
Hashimoto thyroiditis, 70
Helix, 16
Hemizygous, 50
Heterochromatin, 95
Heteroploid, 122
Heterozygous, 46
Histocompatibility, 65
Histone, 21, 89
Hodgkin's disease, 119
Homograft, 65
Homozygous, 46
Hybrid (F$_1$), 38, 43, 45, 66
H-2 gene, 65

Identical twins, 67
Imines, 132
Immunity, 65
Immunosuppression, 67, 68
Incest, 128
Interphase, 20
Inversion, 101, 109, 131
Iso-chromosome, 102
Isograft, 65
Isologous, 69

Karyotype, 24, 25
Klinefelter's syndrome, 106,
    107, 113, 114, 115

Lactose metabolism, 87–88
Leukaemia, 69, 106, 109, 121,
    124, 125
Linkage, 46
Lipid, 2
Lipoprotein, 64
LSD (lysergic acid
    diethylamide), 125
Lupus erythematosis, 70

Lymphocyte, 67, 68
Lyon's hypothesis, 54
Lysis, 95
Lysosome, 2, 3, 4

Macroglobulinaemia, 109
Malaria, 93
Malphigian tube, 84
Meiosis, 33, 34, 35
Melanin, 58, 74, 75
Messenger RNA, 79, 80, 82, 87
Metacentric, 22, 26
Metaphase, 20
Microcephaly, 110
Micrococcus, 15
Microsome, 3, 4
Mitochondria, 2, 4, 122
Mitomycin, 92
Mitosis, 18, 19
Mongolism, 103, 104, 105, 107
Mosaicism, 96, 113–117
Mucopolysaccharide, 64
Mulattos, 58
Multiple allelism, 59
Muscular dystrophy, 57, 112
Mustard gas, 131, 132
Mutants, 78
Mutation, 77, 87, 90, 93, 127, 131
Myasthenia gravis, 70
Myleran, 132

Neurospora, 72, 87, 90
Nitrous acid, 92, 93
Non-disjunction, 99
Nucleic acid, 9
Nucleolus, 9
Nucleotide, 13, 14
Nucleus, 6, 9

Oligomenorrhea, 109
Operator, 86
Operon, 86
Organelles, 2
Ovum, 33

Pelger anomaly, 129
Peromyscus, 26

Peroxide, 132
Phage, 11
Phenylketonuria (PKU), 74, 94, 132, 133, 135
Philadelphia chromosome (Ph'), 121
Plasmodium, 93
Pleiotropy, 94
Pneumococcus, 10
Polar bodies, 35
Polygene, 57
Polymorphism (chromosomal), 26
Polyploidy, 100
Polytene, 84
Primula, 71
Prophase, 20
Protein, 2, 76, 87
Purine, 13
Pyrimidine, 13

Radiation, 125, 130
Recessive, 38
Repeats, 101
Repressor substance, 86, 87
Retinoblastoma, 112
Rhesus blood group (Rh), 62, 63
Rheumatoid arthritis, 70
Ribosome, 3, 4, 79
RNA (ribonucleic acid), 9, 13, 79

Salivary gland chromosome, 21, 84
Salmonella, 74, 75, 95
Satellite, 22
Schizophrenia, 125
Sclerosis (multiple), 70
Sequence hypothesis, 78
Sex chromatin, 54
Sex chromosome, 23
Sex linkage, 49–51
Sex mosaics, 115
Sex ratio, 55
Shope virus, 135
Sickle cell, 77, 93

Simian virus (SV-40), 123
Somatic mutation, 95
Sperm, 33
Spina bifida, 133
Stem cell, 83
Stem-line, 120
Sturge-Weber's syndrome, 109
Submetacentric, 22
Subtelocentric, 22
Sulphur mustard, 92

Telocentric, 22
Telophase, 20
Tetraploid (4n), 100, 112
Thorotrast, 124–125
Thymine, 13
Thymus, 15, 68
Transduction, 95
Transferrin, 63
Transfer RNA, 79
Translocation, 102, 109, 131
Transplantation, 65–67
Triplet, 80, 82

Triploid (3n), 100, 111, 112
Trisomy, 99, 105, 106
Tumour, 69, 129, 135
Turner's syndrome, 106, 107, 115
Tyrosinosis, 74

Ultraviolet, 27, 92
Uracil, 13

Virus (SV-40), 123, 135
Vitamin, 72

X chromosome, 23, 50, 53, 54, 98, 118
Xg blood group, 53
X-rays, 6, 15, 69, 92, 124, 130–131

Y chromosome, 23, 50, 53, 54, 98, 108, 117, 118

Zygote, 46